Nephrology

Editor

SHERRY RIVERA

CRITICAL CARE NURSING CLINICS OF NORTH AMERICA

www.ccnursing.theclinics.com

Consulting Editor
DEBORAH GARBEE

December 2022 • Volume 34 • Number 4

ELSEVIER

1600 John F. Kennedy Boulevard • Suite 1800 • Philadelphia, Pennsylvania, 19103-2899

http://www.theclinics.com

CRITICAL CARE NURSING CLINICS OF NORTH AMERICA Volume 34, Number 4
December 2022 ISSN 0899-5885, ISBN-13: 978-0-323-93959-1

Editor: Kerry Holland
Developmental Editor: Ann Gielou M. Posedio

Critical Care Nursing Clinics of North America (ISSN 0899-5885) is published quarterly by Elsevier Inc., 360 Park Avenue South, New York, NY 10010-1710. Months of issue are March, June, September, and December. Business and Editorial Offices: 1600 John F. Kennedy Blvd., Suite 1800, Philadelphia, PA 19103-2899. Periodicals postage paid at New York, NY and additional mailing offices. Subscription prices are $160.00 per year for US individuals, $593.00 per year for US institutions, $100.00 per year for US students and residents, $206.00 per year for Canadian individuals, $611.00 per year for Canadian institutions, $230.00 per year for international individuals, $611.00 per year for international institutions, $115.00 per year for international students/residents and $100.00 per year for Canadian students/residents. To receive student/resident rate, orders must be accompanied by name of affiliated institution, data of term, and the *signature* of program/residency coordinator on institution letterhead. Orders will be billed at individual rate until proof of status is received. Foreign air speed delivery is included in all *Clinics* subscription prices. All prices are subject to change without notice. **POSTMASTER:** Send address changes to *Critical Care Nursing Clinics of North America*, Elsevier Health Sciences Division, Subscription Customer Service, 3251 Riverport Lane, Maryland Heights, MO 63043. **Customer Service: 1-800-654-2452 (US and Canada); 314-447-8871 (outside US and Canada). Fax: 314-447-8029. E-mail:** JournalsCustomerService-usa@elsevier.com **(for print support) and** JournalsOnlineSupport-usa@elsevier.com **(for online support).**

Reprints. For copies of 100 or more of articles in this publication, please contact the Commercial Reprints Department, Elsevier Inc., 360 Park Avenue South, New York, New York, 10010-1710; Tel.: 212-633-3874, Fax: 212-633-3820, and E-mail: reprints@elsevier.com.

Critical Care Nursing Clinics of North America is covered in *MEDLINE/PubMed (Index Medicus), International Nursing Index, Nursing Citation Index, Cumulative Index to Nursing and Allied Health Literature, and RNdex Top 100.*

Contributors

CONSULTING EDITOR

DEBORAH GARBEE, PhD, APRN, ACNS-BC, FCNS
Associate Dean for Professional Practice, Community Service and Advanced Nursing
Practice, Professor of Clinical Nursing, Louisiana State University Health Sciences Center
New Orleans School of Nursing, New Orleans, Louisiana

EDITOR

SHERRY RIVERA, DNP, APRN, ANP-C, FNKF
Assistant Professor of Clinical Nursing, Adult-Gerontology Primary Care Nurse
Practitioner, Program Coordinator, Louisiana State University Health New Orleans School
of Nursing, New Orleans, Louisiana

AUTHORS

LYN BEHNKE, DNP, FNP-BCBC, PMHNP-BC, CAFCI, FAACPVR, CHFN
Assistant Professor, University of Michigan-Flint, School of Nursing

SUSAN E. BROWN, MS, ARNP, ACNP-BC, CCRN
Southeast Iowa Regional Medical Center—Nephrology, West Burlington, Iowa

CHRISTINE CORBETT, DNP, APRN, FNP-BC, CNN-NP, FNKF
University Health Truman Medical Center, Kansas City, Missouri

JAN BUENACOSA CRUZ, MSN, MPH, APRN, NP-C, CNN-NP
Rocky Mountain Regional VA Medical Center, Aurora, Colorado

LEANNE H. FOWLER, DNP, MBA, AGACNP-BC, CNE
Associate Professor of Clinical Nursing, Director of Nurse Practitioner Programs,
Louisiana State University Health New Orleans School of Nursing, New Orleans, Louisiana

KELLI FROST, MS, PA-C
Assistant Professor, Physician Assistant Program, College of Health Professions,
University of Detroit Mercy, Detroit, Michigan

DEBRA J. HAIN, PhD, APRN, AGPCNP-BC, FAAN, FAANP, FNKF
Professor (Tenured), DNP Program Director, Graduate Co-Coordinator AGNP
Concentration, Florida Atlantic University, Christine E Lynn College of Nursing,
Boca Raton, Florida

MARY S. HARAS, PhD, MBA, APRN, NP-C, CNN
Associate Professor, School of Nursing, Georgetown University, Washington, DC

VIVIAN HEMMAT, MSN, AGACNP-BC, ACHPN
University Health Truman Medical Center, Kansas City, Missouri

M.J. HENDERSON, MS, RN, GNP-BC (retired)
Gerontological Nursing Consultant

KIMBERLY HORKA, AGPCNP-BC
Masters Degree Adult Primary Care Nurse Practitioner, Gerontology Certified, South Lyon, Michigan

KATERINA M. JONES, DNP, APRN, ANP-C, CNN-NP
Metrolina Nephrology Associates, Charlotte, North Carolina

KEVIN M. LOWE, MSN, APRN, ACNP-BC, CNN-NP
Metrolina Nephrology Associates, Charlotte, North Carolina

CATHY MCATEE, DNP, ACNP-BC, CNE
Instructor of Clinical Nursing, Louisiana State University Health New Orleans School of Nursing, New Orleans, Louisiana

CLAIR MILLET, DNP, APRN, PHCNS-BC
Director, Nursing Continuing Professional Development, Assistant Professor of Clinical Nursing, Robert Wood Johnson Foundation Public Health Nurse Leader, Louisiana State University Health New Orleans School of Nursing, New Orleans, Louisiana

BECKY M. NESS, PA-C, MPAS, FNKF, DFAPPA
Instructor of Medicine, Mayo Clinic College of Medicine, Mayo Clinic Health System SWMN Region—Mankato, Mankato, Minnesota

SAMUEL REALISTA
Nurse Practitioner and NP Preceptor, Real Health America LLC, Orlando, Florida

SHERRY RIVERA, DNP, APRN, ANP-C, FNKF
Assistant Professor of Clinical Nursing, Adult-Gerontology Primary Care Nurse Practitioner, Program Coordinator, Louisiana State University Health New Orleans, School of Nursing, New Orleans, Louisiana

Contents

> Medications are a common cause of injury to the kidney and can contribute to the increased progression of disease, poorer outcomes, and increased health care costs. Improved prescribing practices can decrease the risk for the development of acute kidney injury and the progression to end-stage kidney disease. KDIGO Clinical Practice Guidelines recommend the use of caution when prescribing potentially nephrotoxic medications for patients with kidney disease. More than 50–72% of individuals across all stages of kidney disease utilized potentially nephrotoxic medications contributing to poorer outcomes. Annually, 1.5 million adverse drug events causing medication-induced nephrotoxicity occur in the US. Medication-induced nephrotoxicity accounts for 14–26% of cases of AKI in adults and 16% of hospitalized children. It is imperative that nurses and all health care providers are practicing nephrotoxic stewardship to prevent medication-induced nephrotoxicity.

> This article seeks to inform the reader about the global burden of hypertension and highlight the need for therapies to reduce societal costs and mortality associated with hypertension. Hypertension is a worldwide health concern for which international and European evidence and guidelines should be incorporated with the high-quality evidence that has been generated and synthesized in the United States.

> Cardiorenal syndromes (CRS) describe disorders effecting critically ill and hospitalized patients with concurrent heart and kidney dysfunction. The presence of CRS is associated with a poor prognosis. This article is a review of the epidemiology, pathology, and evidence-based evaluation and management strategies for cardiorenal syndromes. All nurses should understand the significance that chronic heart and kidney disease has upon a patient's risk for CRS. Registered and advanced practice nurses should maintain the knowledge and skills of understanding the pathology of CRS to improve the evaluation and management of patients who present with CRS.

Chronic kidney disease (CKD) is a widespread condition that predisposes patients to a myriad of complications, including cardiovascular disease, electrolyte and acid–base derangements, anemia, mineral–bone disease, and volume excess. The frequency of CKD complications increases with the stage of disease, becoming nearly ubiquitous in later stages. The complications of CKD have profound implications for patient management, laboratory monitoring, medication prescribing, and follow up. Management of CKD seeks to slow disease progression and mitigate the risks posed by these complications.

Volume overload is a common complication of a multitude of disease states, as well as a complication of many medical therapies. For the critically ill patient in the intensive care unit, volume overload is especially concerning when persistent past the first few days of admission. In the setting of chronic kidney disease, the maintenance of fluid balance presents additional challenges. This article focuses on the causes of volume overload as well as treatment options of the critically ill patient, including the nuances of the kidney patient, and ends with outpatient guidelines and recommendations to avoid recurrence.

Older adults receiving critical care have a high risk for acute kidney injury (AKI) for many reasons. It is important that critical care nurses know and have the skills to address the risk factors, conduct a comprehensive geriatric assessment, and implement evidence-based interventions. This article provides a review of this information.

The incidence and prevalence of inpatient acute kidney injury is continuing to increase. Acute kidney injury (AKI) is an all-encompassing topic in renal care as well as critical care. The definition and criteria for diagnosis of AKI have evolved over time. There are many causes of AKI and identifying the cause is key in reversing and controlling the progression of disease. Metabolic acidosis, fluid overload, and sepsis require detailed evaluation to best provide the most appropriate plan and execution. Critical care nurses are vitally important when identifying and managing acute kidney injury. Renal replacement therapy is a remarkable tool that requires expertise from the critical nurse. Once it is mastered, the most vulnerable patient in the ICU can become the recipient of good and positive outcomes.

This article provides fundamental information to health care providers on kidney transplant. It reviews some of the preoperative testing, postoperative complications, and treatments. It is to help those who help assist with post-operative care of kidney transplants ensure care is optimal. This article will help educate and inform caregivers of guidelines and suggested plans of care to follow for best outcomes for transplant recipients. The short- and long-term care of these patients are extremely important, and health care providers need to follow practice guidelines to achieve optimal outcomes. This discussion will benefit anyone who has direct care to transplant recipients including, but not limited to: nursing staff, nurses aids, training physicians, general practitioners, and mid-level providers.

Onco-nephrology focuses on the care of patients with cancer and kidney disease. Patients with acute kidney injury, tumor lysis syndrome, and malignancy-associated hypercalcemia are frequently treated in a critical care setting. Oncological emergencies can have a high mortality rate when not promptly recognized and appropriately treated. The critical care nurse should be knowledgeable regarding the risk factors, clinical manifestations, and laboratory abnormalities of common renal manifestations of malignancy and oncological emergencies to optimize care and improve patient outcomes.

Both nephrologists and palliative care specialists are frequently consulted on patients admitted to the intensive care unit suffering from both acute kidney injury and end-stage kidney disease. Dialysis continues to be the predominant treatment recommendation for kidney failure despite the aging population and increased incidence of comorbid conditions. Research shows patients request prognostic information and dialysis survival rates before initiating treatment; however, many patients initiate dialysis naive of their increased morbidity and mortality. Palliative care, in collaboration with nephrology, can help improve communication and a focus on shared decision making.

The COVID-19 pandemic disproportionately affected individuals with kidney disease causing significant morbidity and mortality worldwide. Sars-coV-2 infection has been linked to the development of acute kidney injury and worsening of underlying kidney function. Multiple challenges were encountered during the COVID-19 pandemic resulting in valuable lessons learned for future pandemics, public health emergencies, and disasters related to the care of individuals with kidney disease. The COVID-19 pandemic has further exposed the extensive need for more nurses to be knowledgeable about the care of kidney disease and able to provide specialized nephrology care.

The need for a workforce able to address the health care needs of older adults has been well established. Individuals with kidney disease experience an extensive number of transitions of care across health care settings related to the kidney disease process and the number of health care providers involved in their care. Kidney disease is multifactorial, and the prevention of progression of disease and poor outcomes are key to improving the health of individuals with kidney disease. Nurses and nurse practitioners can improve the outcomes for individuals with complex comorbid conditions and kidney disease especially during the transitions of care.

CRITICAL CARE NURSING
CLINICS OF NORTH AMERICA

SERIES OF RELATED INTEREST

Nursing Clinics of North America http://www.nursing.theclinics.com

THE CLINICS ARE AVAILABLE ONLINE!
Access your subscription at:
www.theclinics.com

Preface

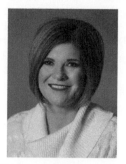

Sherry Rivera, DNP, APRN, ANP-C, FNKF
Editor

Kidney disease is a worldwide public health issue that can affect individuals of all ages, races, ethnicities, and socioeconomic status. Approximately 10% of the population worldwide and 15% in the United States have chronic kidney disease. Research has revealed that health care providers and patients have a lack of awareness about kidney disease. According to the National Kidney Foundation, approximately 90% of individuals with kidney disease lack awareness of their disease status.

Underserved populations experience kidney disease at higher rates than other population groups as witnessed during the COVID-19 pandemic. Many individuals who were infected with the SARS-CoV-2 virus developed acute kidney injury requiring dialysis. The long-term effects of kidney disease related to COVID-19 infection remain to be seen. Early recognition of risk and disease can improve health outcomes and delay progression of disease.

Nurses are the most trusted health care professional and provide care for patients with acute, chronic, and end-stage kidney disease across the lifespan in all health care settings. Nurses are on the front line for providing care and have the ability to provide high-quality, evidence-based care to individuals with kidney disease, ultimately improving patient outcomes. During the COVID-19 pandemic, the shortage of nurses specializing in nephrology became more apparent due to the increased need for acute hemodialysis and continuous renal replacement therapies. Nurses that are knowledgeable about kidney disease can increase patient awareness and improve the health outcomes of individuals with kidney disease. The nephrology nursing workforce needs to be expanded to address the growing needs of the population.

This issue of *Critical Care Nursing Clinics of North America* is dedicated to nephrology topics that are frequently encountered when providing care for individuals with kidney disease and are pertinent to nurses across every health care setting. The topics included cover acute and chronic kidney disease, transplantation, hypertension, the complications of kidney disease, the principles of safe prescribing, and the

Crit Care Nurs Clin N Am 34 (2022) xi–xii
https://doi.org/10.1016/j.cnc.2022.09.001
0899-5885/22/© 2022 Published by Elsevier Inc.

ccnursing.theclinics.com

prevention of medication-induced nephrotoxicity, onconephrology, geriatric nephrology, cardiorenal syndrome, management of fluid overload, transitions of care, shared decision making, palliative care, and conservative medical management.

Sherry Rivera, DNP, APRN, ANP-C, FNKF
Louisiana State University Health New Orleans
School of Nursing
1900 Gravier Street, Room 4A6
New Orleans, LA 70112, USA

Principles for the Prevention of Medication-Induced Nephrotoxicity

Sherry Rivera, DNP, APRN, ANP-C, FNKF

KEYWORDS

- Nephrotoxic medications • Kidney disease • Acute kidney injury
- Chronic kidney injury • Medication-induced kidney disease

KEY POINTS

- Many commonly used medications are potentially nephrotoxic.
- The presence of kidney disease heightens an individual's risk for adverse drug events.
- Medication errors are common and can cause acute kidney injury and/or worsen chronic kidney disease.
- Approximately 14–26% of cases of AKI in adults and 16% of hospitalized children hospitalized are attributed to medication-induced nephrotoxicity.

INTRODUCTION

Approximately 15% of adults in the United States have kidney disease[1] The Kidney Disease Improving Global Outcomes (KDIGO) Clinical Practice Guidelines for the Evaluation and Management of Chronic Kidney Disease strongly recommend that providers use cautious prescribing when utilizing potentially nephrotoxic medications for patients with kidney disease, especially with an estimated glomerular filtration rate of less than 60 mL/min/1.73 m^2.[1,2] The risk for harm versus benefit should be evaluated on an individual basis and potentially nephrotoxic medications should be avoided with safer treatment alternatives considered in the presence of kidney disease. The use of potentially nephrotoxic medications in the presence of kidney disease has been consistently demonstrated in studies despite evidence-based recommendations. According to Kurani and colleagues[1] (2019) and Davis-Ajami and colleagues[3] (2016), more than 50–72% of individuals across all stages of kidney disease utilized potentially nephrotoxic medications contributing to poorer outcomes. The use of potentially nephrotoxic medications can cause medication-induced nephrotoxicity which increases an individual's risk for acute kidney injury, reduced kidney function, and permanent loss of kidney function.

Louisiana State University Health New Orleans, School of Nursing, 1900 Gravier Street, Room 4A6, New Orleans, LA 70112, USA
E-mail address: Srive4@lsuhsc.edu

Crit Care Nurs Clin N Am 34 (2022) 361–371
https://doi.org/10.1016/j.cnc.2022.08.005
0899-5885/22/© 2022 Elsevier Inc. All rights reserved.

In the United States (US), medication errors cause 7000 to 9000 deaths and contribute to more than $40 billion dollars annually.[4] The presence of kidney disease also heightens an individual's risk for adverse drug events. Adverse drug events are linked to causing medication-induced nephrotoxicity. Approximately 1.5 million adverse drug events causing medication-induced nephrotoxicity occur in the US annually and are associated with more than $3.5 billion dollars.[3] Medication-induced nephrotoxicity is linked to the development and progression of chronic kidney disease (CKD) and acute kidney injury (AKI). Annually, 14–26% of cases of AKI in adults and 16% of hospitalized children hospitalized are attributed to medication-induced nephrotoxicity.[5] Older adults and individuals with multiple comorbid conditions are increasingly affected. Among Medicare beneficiaries the rate of first hospitalization with AKI increased by 42% between 2009 and 2019.[6]

It is imperative that nurses and all health care providers are practicing nephrotoxic stewardship to prevent medication-induced nephrotoxicity. All health care providers need to become aware of the presence of kidney disease or risk for development, be familiar with potentially nephrotoxic agents, ensure that appropriate medications are selected, dosing is evaluated, and the potential for drug interactions identified to assist with the preservation of kidney function. Nephrotoxic stewardship can reduce adverse outcomes for individuals with kidney disease.

Potentially nephrotoxic agents

The kidneys are responsible for the filtration, metabolism, and excretion of most medications which heightens the risk for damage to the kidneys. In addition, many commonly used agents such as over the counter and prescribed medications, diagnostic agents, and environmental factors can be potentially nephrotoxic which can heighten the risk for the development of AKI or progression of CKD (**Table 1**).

Exposure to a potentially nephrotoxic medication does not always equate to the development of kidney disease for every individual. However, one medication-related complication occurs for every 2.7 medication exposures among individuals with end-stage kidney disease (ESKD) receiving hemodialysis.[7]

Medication-induced kidney disease is related to a combination of factors such as the potential nephrotoxicity of the agent/medication, length of exposure to the nephrotoxic agent/medication, individual characteristics of the agent/medication, a patient's individual risk factors, and the pharmacokinetic and pharmacodynamic properties of the medication. For injury to occur a combination of these factors is present.[5] Individuals that are vulnerable such as children and older adults may have less muscle mass, and multiple comorbid conditions placing them at a higher risk for AKI and/or progression of CKD.

Adverse drug reactions

Adverse drug reactions (ADRs) are preventable with serious consequences for individuals with kidney disease. Multiple factors contribute to the development of ADRs in the population with kidney disease. A lack of awareness of kidney disease exists due to barriers at the patient, provider, and systemic level and can contribute to an increased risk for medication-induced kidney disease. According to Kurani and colleagues (2019), a cross-sectional analysis of the National Health and Nutrition Examination Surveys (2011–2016) was conducted and demonstrated that 91.6% of adults with CKD stages 3–5 were unaware of having kidney disease. Given the complexity of kidney disease and the risk for complications, efforts to reduce the risk for medication-

Table 1
Potentially nephrotoxic agents (not all inclusive)

Medications	Herbal/Dietary Supplements	Diagnostic Agents	Environmental
Nonsteroidal Anti-inflammatory Medications (NSAIDs)	Aristolochic Acid	Radiocontrast	Lead
	Ephedra	High Dose Gadolinium	Arsenic
Proton Pump Inhibitors	Flavonoid	Colonoscopy Prep	Cadmium
Angiotensin Converting Enzyme Inhibitor (ACE inhibitors)	Bee Pollen		Mercury
	Chromium Picolinate		Copper
	Hawthorn		Bismuth
Angiotensin Receptor Blocker (ARB)	Yellow Oleander		Hydrocarbons
	Licorice		Silicon
Statins	Cat's Claw		Germanium
Acetazolamide	Willow Bark		
Benzodiazepines	Yohimbine		
Beta lactams	Creatine Monohydrate		
Acyclovir	L-Lysine		
Cephalosporin	Chaparral		
Cimetidine	Tripterygium wilfordii hook F (Thunder God Vine)		
Allopurinol	Ascorbic Acid		
Clopidogrel	Vaccinium Macrocarpon		
Methadone	Artemisia absinthium		
Methotrexate	Hydralazine Sulfate		
Aspirin			
Cocaine			
Cortisone			
Amitriptyline			
Cyclophosphamide			
Penicillin			
Aminoglycosides			
Tacrolimus			
Furosemide			
Haloperidol			
Lithium			
Phenytoin			
Probenecid			
Quinolones			
Rifampin			
Vancomycin			
Sulfonamides			

related adverse events are vitally important. An estimated glomerular filtration of less than 30 mL/min per 1.73 m,[2] 3 or more comorbid conditions, polypharmacy with 5 or more medications, changes in medication regimens four times or more within the past year, use of medications that require monitoring, diabetes, chronic kidney disease, and poor adherence with taking prescribed medications increases an individual's risk for ADRs. The perfect storm for ADRs exists when these multiple factors are present in combination. A study conducted by Laville and colleagues[8] (2020), concluded that 40% of ADRs are caused by renin–angiotensin system inhibitors, diuretics, and antithrombotic medications. Adverse drug reactions can be classified as those that cause damage to the kidneys, are complications of kidney disease, or related to omission of therapy. Additional medication-related problem categories can include when the drug is administered without indication, inappropriate drug selection, subtherapeutic dose, overdose, failure to receive the drug, and inappropriate lab monitoring.

A hypersensitivity reaction to medications is an unintended ADR. The term "drug allergy" is often used as a term applied to describe all types of ADRs. Differentiating an ADR from a true hypersensitivity reaction is important. A hypersensitivity reaction to a medication is characterized by the presence of immunologic manifestations such as rash, urticaria, and anaphylaxis with no other identifiable explanation.[9] The onset of symptoms usually occurs within 7–10 days of initial exposure to the medication.[9] With reexposure to the offending agent, symptoms occur within 4 days and are often a more severe presentation.[9] A maculopapular rash with eosinophilia and fever that is new in onset is also indicative of a drug-induced hypersensitivity reaction.[9] A decline in renal function, electrolyte abnormalities, and sterile pyuria may be pertinent contributory laboratory findings.[9]

Medication-induced interstitial nephritis often occurs due to a hypersensitivity or an allergic reaction.[10] The prevalence of antibiotic-induced interstitial nephritis is 78% in developed countries.[10] Seventy to 90 (70–90%) percent of cases identified with kidney biopsy are related to medications.[10] The most common medications that are linked to the development of medication-induced interstitial nephritis include nonsteroidal anti-inflammatory drugs (NSAIDs), proton pump inhibitors (PPIs), and antibiotics. Beta-lactam antibiotics are one of the main causes and can cause rash, eosinophilia, and/or fever within days to weeks of initiating treatment.[10] Approximately 17% of individuals treated with methicillin develop interstitial nephritis.[10] The onset of medication-induced interstitial nephritis from NSAIDs may not be apparent for 6 to 12 months.[10] Onset of PPI-induced interstitial nephritis may occur within one week to 18 months of initiating treatment.[10] Loop, thiazide, and potassium-sparing diuretics are also linked to interstitial nephritis. Presentation of symptoms related to diuretics occurs within 4–10 weeks of initiating treatment.[10] The incidence of medication-induced interstitial nephritis is rising among older adults. Discontinuing the offending agent usually results in the improvement of kidney function; however, return to baseline kidney function only occurs in 30–70% of patients.[10] Chronic interstitial nephritis can occur with continued use of the medication. Inflammation and scarring of renal tissues can develop within 7–10 days and withdrawal of the medication or treatment with steroids may or may not result in improvement.[10] The treatment of acute interstitial nephritis should include withdrawal of the offending agent and administration of corticosteroids for at least one month.[11]

Medications can also damage the glomerular tissue as well. There are 3 main types including injury to the visceral epithelial cell or podocyte, endothelial cells, and mesangial cells.[12] Commonly prescribed medications that have been linked to injury to the glomerular tissues include bisphosphonates, NSAIDs, lithium, sirolimus, antiplatelets, antiangiogenetic medications, and interferon.[12] Patients with medication-induced glomerular disease often present with hematuria, proteinuria, and a reduction in renal function.[12] Recovery of kidney function is dependent upon provider recognition and withdrawal of the offending agent.[12] Close observation is the best method for the identification of this condition.

Individuals with kidney disease are at a higher risk for experiencing adverse drug events or nephrotoxicity than individuals with normal kidney function.[13] Individuals with kidney disease have multiple comorbid conditions and are prescribed numerous medications as treatment of those conditions. Individuals with CKD prescribed an average of 6 to 12 medications.[13] With advancing stages of kidney disease, the average number of medications prescribed increases. By the time an individual has reached end-stage renal disease (ESRD), the median number of medications increases to 19 pills per day.[13] Individuals with kidney disease have higher rates of adverse drug reactions than those with normal kidney function.[13]

Medication Assessment

The treatment of kidney disease is complex. Nurses should be aware that an individual has kidney disease or risk factors for the development of kidney disease, and knowledge about the pharmacokinetic and pharmacodynamic properties of medications. Nurses and other health care providers must ensure that kidney function is evaluated when medications are prescribed for a patient. Evaluating the underlying comorbid conditions, conducting medication reconciliation, evaluating the properties of the medication, and adjusting medication dosage to the degree of renal disease is important when prescribing medications.[14] Safe prescribing in the presence of kidney disease should include the following key components: adhering to prescribing guidelines, conducting a medication assessment and reconciliation, selecting medications based on evidence-based recommendations, adjusting dosing to the degree of kidney disease based on pharmacokinetics and pharmacodynamics, monitoring the kidney function, and evaluating the individual patient's response (**Table 2**).

Evaluating the potential risk and benefits of medications presents medical decision-making challenges. Risks could include the development of ADRs and/or worsening kidney function. It is imperative that providers are frequently evaluating medications and adjusting the dosage as warranted. Episodes of AKI are commonly characterized by rapid changes in kidney function requiring close monitoring and frequent dosing adjustments, whereas CKD may be characterized by a slow progression and less frequent adjustments in dosing.

Deprescribing is also an important aspect of safe prescribing in the presence of kidney disease. Deprescribing is the systematic process of identifying medications that the potential harms outweigh the potential risks. NSAIDs should be deprescribed due to risks for the development of AKI, worsening of underlying kidney disease, hyperkalemia, hypertension, and fluid retention.[14] The potential risks versus the benefits of PPIs use should also be evaluated and considered for deprescribing. Risk factors and current medication use should be evaluated on an individual basis when making deprescribing decisions. Chronic kidney disease can alter the pharmacokinetic or pharmacodynamic properties of medications which can lead to toxicity. The volume of distribution of water-soluble medications can be altered by edema, chronic kidney disease, chronic liver disease, and medications.[14] Evaluating the response to a medication includes monitoring for toxicity and/or drug levels as pertinent.[14]

Over-the-counter medications (OTC), dietary supplements, vitamins, and herbals should also be evaluated. Research is limited regarding the impact that many supplements, vitamins, and herbal substances have in the presence of kidney disease. The National Kidney Foundation's website (https://www.kidney.org/atoz/content/vitamineral) offers a resource to patients, families, and providers regarding many commonly used herbals, supplements, vitamins, and OTC medications.[15] The Natural Medicine Comprehensive Database is also another available resource.[14]

Clinical Pharmacokinetic Considerations

Pharmacokinetics include the absorption, distribution, metabolism, transport, and excretion properties of a medication.[16] Pharmacokinetics properties include the amount of the medication that reaches the site of action. The pharmacokinetics of many medications are altered by kidney disease. Changes in pharmacokinetics in the presence of kidney disease can contribute to over or underdosing of medications increasing the risk for ADR or failure of treatment.[17] It is important that all health care providers are knowledgeable about the basic pharmacokinetic principles when providing care to individuals

Table 2	
Principles for medication assessment	
Step	**Comments**
Assessment of Kidney Function	• Evaluated kidney function using the eGFR and other available labs.
Obtain Medication History	• Conduct a thorough and accurate medication history including over-the-counter medications, dietary supplements, and prescribed medications. • Evaluate medication allergies, medication intolerances, prior episodes of AKI, adjustments to medication regimen due to impaired kidney function.
Conduct a Medication Review	• Evaluate the indication for the medication and necessity. • Assess the dosing and frequency of each medication. • Determine if each medication taken is nephrotoxic or contraindicated due to the degree of kidney function (AKI, chronic kidney disease, end-stage renal disease). • Is the medication or medication's metabolite prolonged in chronic kidney disease? • Ensure appropriate monitoring is being conducted. • Assess adherence and reasons for lack of adherence. • Address any discrepancies in the medical record.
Adjust Medications as Needed	• Utilize medication labeling, information, peer-reviewed literature available. • Collaborate with a pharmacist. • Deprescribe medications one at a time. • Evaluate risks versus benefits. • Identify patient preferences and document preferences. • Communicate with all members of the health care team.
Medication Monitoring Considerations	• Adapt the medication plan depending on if there are acute or chronic changes in health or kidney status? Is there a decline or improvement in the patient's status? • Monitor medications appropriately according to recommendations if pertinent. • Document medication changes, regimens, pertinent information, especially any changes in status or symptoms and if a medication was initiated or discontinued.

Adapted from Whittaker CF, Miklich MA, Patel RS, Fink JC. (2018). Medication Safety Principles and Practice in CKD. Clin J Am Soc Neph, 13: 1738-1746.

with kidney disease. Prescribing for and/or administering medications to individuals with kidney disease requires knowledge about the individual medication, the alterations in physiology that occur due to kidney disease, and the pharmacokinetic principles that may impact dosing regimens. The ability to apply pharmacokinetic principles is especially helpful when the case is complicated or when guidance is limited. The prescriber and the nurses administering the medication also need to be aware of the multiple factors that can impact how the medication is handled. When appropriate dosing is uncertain starting "low and going slow" is a commonly used approach; however, this approach may be less beneficial when the rapid onset of the medication is desired.[17] The therapeutic target, initial dose, maintenance dose, frequency of dose, and timing of dose adjustments are key principles for consideration when prescribing.[17]

Table 3
Pharmacokinetic properties and AKI, CKD, and renal replacement therapies

Pharmacokinetic Property	AKI	CKD	Renal Replacement Therapy (RRT)
Absorption	Decrease possible	Increase or decrease possible	Limited effect
Volume of Distribution	No change to increase possible	No change to increase possible	Decrease possible to no change
Metabolism	Difficult to determine, CYP3A4/5 may decrease	Decreased clearance	Increase following treatment for the unknown period or quantity possible
Excretion	Kidney: decreased, rapid changes, dependent on severity Nonkidney: difficult to determine	Kidney: stable to decreased Nonkidney: possible decreased, difficult to determine	Kidney: unchanged Nonkidney: difficult to determine
Elimination	Decrease or increase possible		Increased removal of medication (dependent on the medication, type of RRT, duration, and dialysis prescription)

Adapted from Roberts DM, Sevastos J, Carland JE, Stocker SL, Lea-Henry TN. (2018). Clinical Pharmacokinetics in Kidney Disease to Rational Design of Dosing Regimens. Clin J Am Soc Neph, 13: 1254-1263.

To reduce the risk related to medications in the presence of kidney disease, the calculation of creatinine clearance has been utilized for decades. There have been multiple equations developed over time to assist with calculating the creatinine clearance; however, each equation has its own unique set of challenges, limitations, and benefits. Prescribing applications have been developed to assist with this process making the information more readily available and easily accessible to the clinician.

The inclusion of the estimated glomerular filtration rate (eGFR) in basic and comprehensive metabolic panel results has also widely increased access to valuable information that can be used for staging kidney disease and dosing medications. Challenges remain regarding the use of eGFR for medication dosing adjustment related to race, age, weight, acuity of illness, and muscle mass demonstrating the need for additional research and the need for clinical interpretation to be individualized. There has also been debate regarding the equation utilized to calculate the eGFR for medication dosing; however, research has demonstrated that the dose of medication remained the same regardless of the equation utilized.[18] It is important to recognize that medication dosing decisions should be made with clinical judgment and consideration of individual patient factors, not just the eGFR.

Kidney disease consists of a heterogenous group of conditions that differ in severity and impact the kidney in a variety of areas such as the vasculature, tubulointerstitium, and glomeruli and alters pharmacokinetic properties.[17] There is variability among the types and severity of kidney disease which can impact medication clearance, but this is difficult to quantify with limited research available. Due to a lack of research, medication dosing recommendations are inconsistent and may not be applicable to every type of kidney disease.[17] When making clinical decisions it is important to consider the primary purpose of the medication, the goal of use, risks versus benefits, the initial dose, frequency of dosing, maintenance dosing, and when dosing should be adjusted, individual patient risk factors, disease-related factors, acuity and severity of illness, and treatment type. For example, the absorption of medications from the gastrointestinal tract can be variable among individuals with CKD (**Table 3**).[17]

Medication dosing adjustments are complex in AKI due to the multiple physiologic changes that occur affecting volume status and organ dysfunction. Critical illness can also affect the absorption of medications.[17] CKD and AKI are different conditions with differing effects on pharmacokinetic properties and require knowledge of the individual concepts of pharmacokinetics. A decline in eGFR occurs in AKI, CKD, and ESRD and decreases medication clearance through the kidney. The volume of distribution may remain the same or increase.[19] Fluid overload is more likely to impact the volume of distribution of hydrophilic medications than lipophilic medications. Uremia can cause altered volume of distribution of protein-bound medication.[14] Kidney disease can cause impairment of drug absorption by the gastrointestinal tract due to alterations in gastric pH or edema.[14] Roberts and colleagues[17] (2018) report that a practical method for approaching medication dosing is to assume that medication clearance through the kidney will decrease in proportion to the eGFR and that nonrenal clearance will remain unchanged.

Medication clearance by renal replacement therapies can also be challenging and should be considered for the timing of medication dosing and when adjusting dosing. Information about the effect of dialysis on the clearance of medications is often lacking. The Dialysis of Drugs Publication reports that only 10% of currently utilized medications have reports for dialytic clearance.[20] With intermittent dialysis administering medications following dialysis is possible but becomes more challenging with continuous renal replacement therapies. Data are even more limited with regard to the impact of drug clearances during CRRT. Individual prescription variables such as rates of ultrafiltration, blood, and dialysate can also contribute to significant variability in drug clearances. Blood flow rates affect the clearance rates of drugs and solutes during CRRT to a greater extent. As such, precise prescriptive techniques are difficult to recommend due to the multiple variables and limited availability of data.

When available, therapeutic drug monitoring can be a useful tool to assist with optimizing medication dosing but comes with limitations. Therapeutic drug monitoring can be useful for adjusting treatment depending on if the concentration is outside the desired range or not. This is a key component of antibiotic and nephrotic stewardship. It is important to ensure that the lab sample is drawn at the correct time. A limitation to the practice is that results may have a long turnaround time to be of value within a reasonable time frame. Depending upon the medication, it may be possible to administer a dose midway through the dialysis treatment.

Elimination is the length of time for the plasma concentration to decrease by 50%. The length of time for elimination will double if a decrease in the creatinine clearance by 50% occurs or if the volume of distribution doubles.[19] Failure to adjust the medication dosage in the presence of reduced kidney function will lead to accumulation and toxicity.[19] The medication and its active metabolites can accumulate causing toxic effects such as coma with morphine or seizures from meperidine.[19]

Clinical Pharmacodynamic Considerations

Pharmacokinetics and pharmacodynamics have a cause and consequence relationship. Pharmacodynamics are the consequence of pharmacokinetics. Pharmacodynamics is the effect of a medication on an individual's body, any potential

Table 4
Medication pharmacodynamics

Factors influencing drug concentration at the receptor site
    Medication dosage
    Pharmacokinetics of the medication
    Number of receptors
    Organ's response to the activation of the receptors
    Competing factors at the receptor site
Pathophysiologic Processes that can alter the clinical response
    Aging
    Chronic illnesses
    Kidney disease
    Reduction in number of receptors and sensitivity
    Decreased binding at the receptor site
    Altered transduction
Medications interaction and competition for receptors
    Synergistic effects
    Antagonistic effects
    Medication toxicity

Adapted from Keller F, Hann A. (2018). Clinical Pharmacodynamics Principles of Drug Response and Alterations in Kidney Disease. Clin J Am Soc Neph, 13: 1413-1420.

medication interactions, and its intended target, and any potential biochemical effects ultimately, resulting in the individual's response to the medication.[19] There are 2 different mechanisms involved with pharmacodynamics. The reversible effects and the irreversible effects. Reversible effects include receptor-mediated effects and potential saturation of the medication.[21] Irreversible effects are directly proportional to rising concentrations.[21] Saturation is limited by the total number of binding sites. **(Table 4)**

Acute Kidney Injury Prevention

Acute kidney injury (AKI) is preventable. Critical illness, major surgery, and exposure to nephrotoxic medications can heighten an individual's risk.[22] An assessment of kidney health should be conducted at least annually to determine an individual's AKI risk profile.[22] If exposure occurs, the individual's level of risk should be reevaluated. It is imperative that providers are aware of signs and symptoms of AKI. Assessment of risk factors for AKI should be evaluated during hospitalization including serum creatinine, serum creatinine, urinalysis, and total urine output. Approximately 28% of adverse events leading to AKI are due to nephrotoxic meds.[22] Hospitals and providers should incorporate the concepts of nephrotic stewardship and include a thorough review of medications. Medication-related kidney injury occurs most commonly related to antibiotics, nonsteroidal anti-inflammatory medications (NSAIDs), proton pump inhibitors, antivirals, selective serotonin reuptake inhibitors, chemotherapy, immunosuppressants, and renin–angiotensin–aldosterone system medications. There is an increased risk of being exposed to nephrotoxins in the hospital. The prevalence of exposure to nephrotoxic medications during hospitalization exceeds 75%.[23] For each exposure to a nephrotoxic medication, the risk for AKI increases by 53%.[23]

SUMMARY

The safety of prescribing in the presence of kidney disease is a primary concern. Medications are a common cause of injury to the kidney which can contribute to increased progression of disease, poorer outcomes, and increased health care costs. Improved prescribing can decrease the risk for the development of AKI and progression to end-stage kidney disease.[24] Individuals with kidney disease have multiple comorbid conditions which require great attention to detail when reviewing medications and determining the safety of treatment. Nurses and health care providers need to be aware of potentially nephrotoxic medications and the individual risk factors of their patients and intervene as warranted.

CLINICS CARE POINTS

- KDIGO strongly recommends that providers use caution when prescribing potentially nephrotoxic medications for patients with kidney disease
- Despite evidence-based recommendations for safer prescribing practices in the presence of kidney disease, 50–72% of individuals across all stages of kidney disease are taking potentially nephrotoxic medications.

DISCLOSURE

No disclosures.

REFERENCES

1. Kurani S, Jeffrey MM, Thorsteinsdottir B, et al. Use of potentially nephrotoxic medications by US adults with chronic kidney disease: NHANES, 2011-2016. J Gen Intern Med 2019;35(4):1092–101.
2. Kidney Disease Improving Global Outcomes. Chronic kidney disease evaluation and management. 2012. Available at: https://kdigo.org/guidelines/ckd-evaluation-and-management/. Accessed May 14, 2022.
3. Davis-Ajami ML, Fink JC, Wu J. Nephrotoxic medication exposure in US adults with predialysis chronic kidney disease: health services utilization and cost outcomes. J Manag Care Spec Pharm 2016;22(8):959–68.
4. Tariq RA, Vashisht R, Sinha A, et al. Medication dispensing errors and prevention. 2022. Available at: https://www.ncbi.nlm.nih.gov/books/NBK519065/#_NBK519065_pubdet_. Accessed May 14, 2022.
5. Perazella MA. Pharmacology behind common drug nephrotoxicities. Clin J Am Soc Neph 2018;13:1897–907.
6. United States Renal Data System. 2021 annual report. 2021. Available at: https://adr.usrds.org/2021. Accessed May 14, 2022.
7. Tieu A, House AA, Urquhart BL. Drug disposition issues in CKD: implications for drug discovery and regulatory approval. Adv Chronic Kidney Dis 2016;23(2):63–6.
8. Laville SM, Gras-Champel V, Moragny J, et al. Adverse drug reactions in patients with CKD. Clin J Am Soc Neph 2020;15:1090–102.
9. Raghavan R, Shawar S. Mechanisms of drug-induced interstitial nephritis. Adv Chronic Kidney Dis 2017;24(2):64–71.
10. Nast CC. Medication-induced interstitial nephritis in the 21st Century. Adv Chronic Kidney Dis 2017;24(2):72–9.
11. Moledina DG, Perazella MA. Treatment of drug-induced acute tubulointerstitial nephritis: the search for better evidence. Clin J Am Soc Neph 2018;13:1785–7.
12. Markowitz GS, Bomback AS, Perazella MA. Drug-induced glomerular disease: direct cellular injury. Clin J Am Soc Neph 2015;10:1291–9.

13. Nolin TD, Perazella MA. Introduction to nephropharmacology for the clinician a new CJASN series. Clin J Am Soc Neph 2018;13:1083–4.
14. Whittaker CF, Miklich MA, Patel RS, et al. Medication safety principles and practice in CKD. Clin J Am Soc Neph 2018;13:1738–46.
15. National Kidney Foundation. Vitamins and minerals in chronic kidney disease. 2022. Available at: https://www.kidney.org/atoz/content/vitamineral.
16. Perazella MA, Nolin TD. Adverse drug effects in patients with CKD primum non nocere. Clin J Am Soc Neph 2020;15:1075–7.
17. Roberts DM, Sevastos J, Carland JE, et al. Clinical pharmacokinetics in kidney disease to rational design of dosing regimens. Clin J Am Soc Neph 2018;13:1254–63.
18. Hudson JQ, Nolin TD. Pragmatic use of kidney function estimates for drug dosing: the tide is turning. Adv Chronic Kidney Dis 2018;25(1):14–20.
19. Lea-Henry TN, Carland JE, Stocker SL, et al. Clinical pharmacokinetics in kidney disease fundamental principles. Adv Chronic Kidney Dis 2018;13:1085–95.
20. Tieu A, Velenoski TJ, Kucey AS, et al. beta-blocker dialyzability in maintenance hemodialysis patients. Clin J Am Soc Nephrol 2018;13(4):604–11.
21. Keller F, Hann A. Clinical pharmacodynamics principles of drug response and alterations in kidney disease. Clin J Am Soc Neph 2018;13:1413–20.
22. Kashani K, Rosner MH, Haase M, et al. Quality improvement goals for acute kidney injury. Clin J Am Soc Neph 2019;14:941–53.
23. Martin M, Wilson FP. Utility of electronic medical record alerts to prevent drug nephrotoxicity. Clin J Am Soc Neph 2019;14:115–23.
24. Cardone KE, Bacchus S, Assimon MM, et al. Medication-related problems in CKD. Adv Chronic Kidney Dis 2010;17(5):404–12.

Hypertension

Cathy McAtee, DNP, ACNPC-BC, CNE

KEYWORDS

- Blood pressure • Hypertension • Evidence-based • Guidelines • Monitoring
- Treatment

KEY POINTS

- Hypertension is a global threat to health and is a major contributor to hypertension mediated organ damage such as heart failure, kidney failure, peripheral arterial disease and stroke.
- Hypertension is vastly underdiagnosed and undertreated, even in high income developed countries worldwide.
- Non-pharmacological lifestyle changes are crucial to the prevention and treatment of hypertension.
- Pharmacological therapies that are available are safe and effective for the prevention of the progression of heart failure, kidney failure, peripheral arterial disease.

HYPERTENSION

Hypertension is a major cause of cardiovascular disease worldwide and contributes significantly to the progression of heart failure, renal failure, peripheral arterial disease, and stroke in the adult population. Nearly one in three adults is affected.[1] Hypertension is the second leading cause of kidney disease and can develop as a result of having kidney disease. Hypertension has also been implicated as the causative factor in at least 75% of all heart failure cases.[2] Despite recent advances in awareness and treatment, only half of the population in the United States has blood pressure (BP) readings that are considered well controlled.[3] According to recent research, hypertension is the highest-ranking modifiable risk factor for cardiovascular deaths in the United States.[4] Globally, hypertension is the leading cause of death in adults. A socioeconomic disparity has also been identified in low-to-middle-income countries (LMIC) where there is a reduction both in awareness and treatment.[5]

History

The development and effects of hypertension have been a concept in the making for centuries. As early as 2600 BC, salt intake was identified as a risk factor for the disease

A broad overview of hypertension to includes epidemiology, pathophysiology, diagnostic criteria, and current evidence-based therapy for treatment and monitoring.
Louisiana State University Health Science Center-New Orleans, 1900 Gravier Street, New Orleans LA 70112, USA
E-mail address: cmcat2@lsuhsc.edu

Crit Care Nurs Clin N Am 34 (2022) 373–381
https://doi.org/10.1016/j.cnc.2022.08.002
0899-5885/22/© 2022 Elsevier Inc. All rights reserved.

that was identified as "hard pulses."[6] In 1150 BC, an Egyptian physician was responsible for describing the first temporal relationship between BP and cardiovascular disease. Medieval therapies using acupuncture, venesection, and bleeding by leaches were the earliest known therapies used in history. The concept of measuring BP began in 1733 but had a 95-year hiatus in research until Jean Léonard Marie Poiseuille introduced the mercury manometer as part of his doctoral dissertation. Carl Ludwig made significant improvements to Poiseuille's manometer device and devised the kymograph invasive BP tracings that are, in fact, quite similar to modern-day BP tracings.[6] Before the innovation of electronic transducers, BP was measured in columns of either water or mercury.[7] Noninvasive BP measurement innovations were developed in the early 1900s and were refined by Nicolai Korotkoff in 1905 to include systolic and diastolic BP readings,[6] and hypertension as a clinical entity came about shortly after the sphygmomanometer became available in the early 1900s. Hypertension itself was a disease largely untreated until the 1940s, when President Roosevelt died from complications of uncontrolled hypertension. Pharmacological therapies for hypertension accelerated after World War II, and reserpine, hydralazine, and hydrochlorothiazide were among the first drugs prescribed for chronic hypertension. Today, there is a vast armamentarium of drugs to treat nearly all forms of hypertension, and evidence-based guidelines for their use have been established and refined by the Joint National Commission (JNC), the American College of Cardiology (ACC), and the American Heart Association (AHA). The improvements in the treatment of hypertension have been clinically proven to improve health outcomes in the United States and abroad.[8]

Epidemiology

In the United States, 30% of adult men and 28.1% of adult women are affected by hypertension. As treatment options advanced over the past 50 years, the rates of hypertension declined; however, the progress achieved has since plateaued. The plateau is primarily considered to be caused by an aging population and widespread obesity. Hypertension trends are expected to continue to increase significantly over the next two decades due to rising rates of obesity and an aging population.[9] African American women are most affected at 41.5%, followed by African American men who trail slightly at 40.8%, non-Hispanic whites at 28%, Hispanic Americans at 25.9%, and non-Hispanic Asians at 24.9%. Trends in the United States have been closely monitored through the National Health and Nutrition Study (NHANES), a longitudinal study examining awareness, treatment, and control that provides continuous data collection. According to NHANES data collected from 2012 to 2014, 82.7% of Americans were aware of having hypertension, but only 75.6% were being treated with antihypertensive medications, and only 51.8% had BPs that were considered to be well controlled.

Annually, hypertension accounts for 10.4 million deaths globally. International data suggest that the prevalence of the most severe BPs has shifted from high-income countries (HIC) (349 million) to LMICs (1.04 billion). The disparity noted is secondary to lower levels of awareness, treatment, and control in LMICs. Although initiatives have been implemented to improve awareness, treatment, and management, rates of hypertension are increasing worldwide regardless of income level. The International Society of Hypertension developed updated global hypertension guidelines in 2020 that can be used by both HIC and LMICs by specifying essential and optimal standards of therapy depending on the available resources.[5]

Pathophysiologic Considerations

Short-term regulation of circulatory blood flow involves a complex relationship between local vascular conditions, neurohormonal interactions, and pump mechanics.

Chronic regulation involves additional factors such as volume and vascular capacitance. These systems regulate the BP to maintain an equilibrium between the intake and output of salt and water. Tissues can auto-regulate blood flow and cardiac output (CO) based on their immediate metabolic needs across variable ranges in BP. This homeostatic mechanism maintains flow to the tissues at a normal level despite the increase in total peripheral vascular resistance (TPR) associated with chronic hypertension. Myogenic vasoconstriction can be activated by vascular stretch and hypertension. In most tissues, local vasoconstrictor mechanisms are stimulated if blood flow exceeds the metabolic demands of the tissues. Chronic elevations in BP initiate structural changes that include declining numbers of capillaries and thickening of the arterial vessel walls. Angiotensin II and endothelin often parallel increased TPR and BP, but the flow is generally adequate to meet the tissue's metabolic needs. When the BP is elevated, the blood flow and CO can be maintained by indirect factors in most peripheral tissues except for the kidneys, where optimal BP is essential to maintain glomerular filtration and the excretion of water and electrolytes equivalent to that of intake. For example, renal artery constriction instigates an increase in systemic arterial pressure to compensate and maintain renal perfusion and sodium and water excretion.[10]

The kidney has been recognized as having at least four crucial roles in hypertension. Renin, produced almost exclusively in the kidney's afferent arterioles juxtaglomerular cells, activates the renin–angiotensin system (RAS) by cleaving angiotensinogen and angiotensin I. The release of renin is in response to decreased perfusion pressure, a reduction in sodium delivery to the cells of the macula densa, and increased stimulation of the sympathetic nervous system. Abnormal renin production in the proximal tubule can be seen in conditions of oxidative stress or an increase in the glomerular filtration of protein. The second crucial role of the kidney in influencing hypertension is its ability to regulate circulating volume through diuresis and natriuresis. It will increase diuresis and natriuresis in response to excessive rising BP levels through multiple pathways that include alterations of the sodium hydrogen transporter 3 (NHE3) and the sodium-phosphate cotransporter isoform 2 (NaPi-2a). The translocation of the transporters to the apical microvilli can promote sodium reabsorption in chronic hypertension, which likely further sustains increases in circulating volume and BP. A third function of the kidney is to regulate systemic sympathetic tone through the generation of signaling by the afferent nerves of the kidney. Approximately 10% of the renal nerves are afferent, and 90% are efferent, where these signals increase sodium reabsorption, increase renin release, and enhanced motor tone. Afferent signals initiate reflexes in the brainstem, causing an increase in sympathetic tone, which promotes arterial hypertension. The fourth mechanism of renal influence on hypertension is the immune activation resulting from the migration of antigen-presenting dendritic cells to secondary lymphoid tissue, and the activation of T cells and subsequent antigen formation in angiotensin II (Ang II) induced hypertension. The innate and adaptive immune system plays a vital role in the development of hypertension. Over the past 50 years, research has shown an accumulation of inflammatory cells in the blood vessels and kidneys of hypertensive individuals.[11] Intrarenal T cells are crucial in sustaining hypertension.[12] As these inflammatory cells migrate to the interstitium of the kidney, cytokines are released that have a negative impact on vascular and renal structure and functions[11] as well as the end-organ damage that accompanies hypertension.[11]

In addition to the renal mechanisms described, the vasculature contributes significantly to the development of hypertension. An elevation in systemic vascular resistance can be seen in nearly all cases of hypertension and result from four distinct processes.[11] Thickening and narrowing of the renal arterioles are present in about 98% of all hypertension cases[12] Enhancements of vasoconstrictor hormones such as angiotensin II, vasopressin, and other catecholamines stimulate vasoconstriction. The second mechanism of hypertension is a reduction in nitric oxide (NO) signaling and endothelium-dependent vasodilation with some variability in vessel type. Smaller arteries and arterioles are regulated by endothelium-dependent hyperpolarization and prostaglandins, whereas larger vessels rely on the effects of NO for vasodilation. Impaired synthesis and bioavailability of NO and its cofactors extend beyond the local environment and affect both the central nervous system and renal system to promote hypertension. A second vascular alteration that contributes to hypertension is vascular remodeling. Hypertrophy of the smooth muscle and narrowing of the intravascular lumen directly increases systemic vascular resistance. Remodeling is thought to be secondary to the growth-promoting effects of catecholamines, Ang II, inflammatory cytokines, and oxidative signaling. Oxidative stress has been found to contribute to the development of hypertension, although the exact mechanism is elusive. In the kidney, reactive oxygen species (ROS) oxidatively degrade NO, which in turn increases vasoconstriction and lowers the glomerular filtration rate. Antioxidant therapy thus far has been an ineffective treatment of both cardiovascular disease and hypertension and may remove the beneficial ROS used in normal cell signaling.[13]A third vascular change that likely contributes to hypertension is a stiffening of large conduit arteries such as the aorta. The ability of the aorta to distend and recoil during the cardiac cycle reduces systolic BP while maintaining perfusion and diastolic BP. An increase in pulse wave velocity may indicate aortic stiffening and may be observed years before clinical hypertension occurs. The fourth vascular mechanism contributing to hypertension is a target and source of immune activation, which impairs the vessel wall defenses against thrombosis.[11] The central nervous system influences hypertension through the effect of Ang II neural activation of the sympathetic nervous system. Persons with hypertension have an increase in sympathetic outflow and an amplified response to catecholamine-mediated vasoconstriction. The presence of Ang II and ROS block the vasodilating effect of the microvascular endothelium hyperpolarizing factor.

Aldosterone plays a significant role in kidney hypertension by enhancing sodium resorption in the collecting duct. Mineralocorticoid receptors (MR) have also been discovered in extrarenal sites such as the heart, brain, and blood vessels. An estimated 5% of all hypertensions are due to primary hyperaldosteronism and possibly more with resistant hypertension.[11]

Definition and Diagnostic Criteria

Normal BP: systolic blood pressure (SBP) of <120 mm Hg and a diastolic blood pressure (DBP) <85.

Elevated BP: SBP between 120–129 mm Hg and a DBP <85–89 mm Hg.

Stage I hypertension: SBP 140–159 and/or DBP 90–99 mm Hg.

Stage II hypertension: SBP $\geq$ 160 mm Hg and/or DBP $\geq$ 100 mm Hg.

Resistant BP: >140/90 on a patient who is taking three or more maximally dosed antihypertensive medications, including a diuretic.[5]

Masked hypertension should be considered when BPs appear normal in the office, but ambulatory and/or home measurements are elevated. Masked hypertension commonly affects younger patients, individuals who smoke, male patients, higher alcohol consumption, and higher levels of job stress, and anxiety. White coat hypertension can affect anywhere from 30% to 40% of patients with elevated in-office readings that are normal when checked in ambulatory or home settings. This type of hypertension is seen more in older populations, women, and patients that do not smoke.[14] Accuracy in measurement of BPs is important because pseudo-resistance and white coat hypertension are quite common, BP measurements should occur over 2 or 3 office visits and be confirmed by out-of-office BP readings unless the BP is >180/110 with concurrent evidence of cardiovascular disease. The BP was obtained in a quiet room. Patients should be asked to refrain from smoking or exercise for 30 minutes before measurement, and the bladder should be empty at the time of the evaluation. Using a properly fitted cuff and a validated oscillatory upper arm device, whereas the patient is seated with both feet flat on the floor will improve the quality of the BP readings. Three measurements should be obtained at each visit, with one minute between measurements.[5]

Secondary Hypertension

Secondary causes can be seen in approximately 5% to 10% of all cases of hypertension. Early detection of secondary hypertension accompanied by targeted treatment can cure hypertension in some cases and improve the quality of life for patients with fewer medications and side effects.[5] Screening for secondary hypertension should be performed if the BP is resistant to treatment or if physical examination findings are suggestive of a secondary cause.[4] Common causes of secondary hypertension include renovascular disease, renal parenchymal disease, primary aldosteronism, obstructive sleep apnea (OSA), and drug or alcohol-induced hypertension. Renal ultrasound with duplex Doppler can be used to screen the patient for renal-related causes such as renal artery stenosis, adrenal adenomas, or masses. Renin-to-aldosterone ratio is used to rule out hyperaldosteronism. A thorough sleep history should be obtained and patients at high risk for OSA should be referred for polysomnography. Social history is needed to evaluate for risk of substance-induced hypertension such as tobacco, recreational drugs, and alcohol use. A review of all medications, herbals, and supplements should be conducted. Drugs known to cause hypertension include (but are not limited to) nicotine, nonsteroidal anti-inflammatory drugs, cyclosporin, tacrolimus, oral contraceptives, cocaine, amphetamines, erythropoietic agents, nasal decongestants, and clonidine withdrawal. Less common causes of secondary hypertension occur in less than 1% of cases and include pheochromocytoma, Cushing's syndrome, hypothyroidism, hyperthyroidism, aortic coarctation, primary hyperparathyroidism, congenital adrenal hyperplasia, acromegaly, and other mineralocorticoid excess syndromes.[4]

Discussion

The treatment of hypertension should be based on the guideline-directed evidence-based therapies published in the United States and globally. An extensive review of the literature reveals that high-quality evidence exists for the prevention, detection, clinical evaluation, and treatment of hypertension.[4] Although there are minor variations in hypertension definitions between the Executive Summary of 2017 ACC/AHA, the 2020 International Society of Hypertension Practice Guidelines, and the Kidney Disease Improving Global Outcomes (KDIGO) Clinical Practice Guidelines for Management of Blood Pressure in Chronic Kidney Disease (2021), the underlying recommendations are very similar. The international guidelines consider the lack of resources in LMICs when establishing a realistic plan of care for all countries where hypertension is a significant threat to health.[5]

Lifestyle Modifications

A reduction in the daily intake of sodium has been clinically proven to reduce BP in several clinical trials and is considered a core component of hypertension management. Individuals that are at a higher risk for the development of hypertension should consider a reduction in sodium intake. The most significant benefit of dietary sodium reduction is seen in black Americans, patients living with diabetes and chronic kidney disease, and the older population.[14] A slight reduction in daily sodium intake can prevent thousands of deaths associated with hypertension and billions of dollars in annual health care costs.[15] Average salt intake is variable from country to country and between regions. Still, it is recommended that sodium intake should not exceed 2.0 g/day in the general population, with 80% of daily salt intake derived from hidden food processing sources.[14] The Institute of Medicine recommends a maximum intake of 1500 mg of sodium for most patients.[16] Approximately 40% of the US population with hypertension are obese. Chronic low-grade inflammation, insulin resistance, increased sodium resorption with volume expansion and higher RAAS, and sympathetic activity may be contributing factors to obesity. Weight loss has been clinically proven to reduce the cardiovascular risks associated with hypertension.[15]

Regular physical activity is also beneficial for patients in preventing and treating hypertension.[14] In a study by Lopes and colleagues,[17] aerobic exercise, even at low intensity for older adults, resulted in immediate improvement in SBP of at least 8 mm Hg and has a positive association with chronic reduction of BP over 8 weeks. The exact mechanism for the positive effects of exercise is still unclear but may be due to a reduction in CO, decreased TPR, and decreased sympathetic nervous system and renal–angiotensin activities.[15] The promotion of healthy lifestyle habits should be recommended to all patients with normal BPs and for those with elevated BPs in combination with BP-lowering medications.[4]

Evaluation and Treatment of Hypertension

A clinical evaluation is needed to establish a diagnosis of hypertension, grade the severity, rule out potential secondary causes, and identify contributing factors such as lifestyle, and family history. Proper technique should be reviewed and used when obtaining BP readings to ensure the accuracy of readings. A thorough review of medications should also be conducted to identify potential contributing factors, interactions, and current treatment. The evaluation should include an appraisal of hypertensive mediated organ damage (HMOD) that exists at the time of the evaluation. Key components of the HMOD evaluation should include a neurological examination, fundoscopic examination, auscultation and palpation of the heart, carotids, and peripheral arteries; and BP readings from the right and left arms. Laboratory analysis of the hypertensive patient should include chemistries, complete blood count, fasting lipid profile, hemoglobin A1C, liver function tests, and urinalysis with albumin to creatine ratio. A 12-lead electrocardiogram (EKG) should be performed at this evaluation to evaluate the myocardium's rhythm and potential structural changes.[14] The guide to pharmacological treatment of hypertension should be based on atherosclerotic cardiovascular disease (ASCVD) risk estimation of 10% or higher when the average SBP is > 130 mm Hg and average DBP >80 mm Hg when considering therapy for primary prevention. If ASCVD risk is < 10%, the parameter of 140 mm Hg and DBP > 90 mm Hg can be used. The secondary prevention of recurrent CVD uses the same average parameters of SBP >130 mm Hg and DBP >80.[4]

Five major drug classes are available for first-line therapy, which have been proven to reduce BP. The initial selection may be based on cause-specific differences in cardiovascular outcomes of interest and individual patient factors. Preferential use of drugs for some conditions such as diabetes, stroke, or coronary artery disease (CAD) may predominate the selection from available first-line choices.[14] Diuretic therapy has been the cornerstone of antihypertensive therapy as these drugs were first developed for clinical use. A relative contraindication is the reduced effectiveness in chronic kidney disease (CKD) with an estimated glomerular filtration rate (GFR) < 45 mL/min.[14] First-line therapy with a thiazide or thiazide-type diuretics can lower BP. Chlorthalidone may be the preferred option due to the prolonged half-life and proven reduction in cardiovascular disease. The use of diuretics increases the risk for the development of gout. The presence of gout is a relative contraindication to use unless the patient is on uric acid-reducing therapy. Fluid overload is a common complication related to chronic kidney disease therefore, diuretics are generally beneficial for hypertension management.

Angiotensin-converting enzyme (ACE) or angiotensin receptor blockers (ARBs) can be used in the non-childbearing population but should be avoided in pregnancy. There is a higher risk of hyperkalemia in patients with chronic kidney disease, and a risk of renal failure when bilateral renal artery stenosis is present. Caution must be used when given concurrently with potassium supplements or potassium-sparing diuretics to avoid resultant hyperkalemia. ACE inhibitors are contraindicated persons with a history of angioedema. However, ARB can be used in persons with a history of angioedema 6 weeks after the ACE inhibitor is discontinued.[4] ARBs are better tolerated than other antihypertensive therapies and have a much lower rate of discontinuance related to adverse events. ACE or ARBs are preferred in patients with diabetes and are clinically proven to slow the progression of diabetic and nondiabetic proteinuria and CKD. Both drugs are effective in the prevention and regression of HMOD, such as left ventricular hypertrophy, small vessel remodeling, and the incidence of atrial fibrillation.[14]

Calcium channel blockers (CCBs) are avoided in patients with heart failure with reduced ejection fraction (HFrEF); amlodipine and felodipine can be used if necessary. Pedal edema is a common side effect of CCBs. Pedal edema is more common in female patients and is a dose-related side effect of CCBs. Concurrent use with a beta blocker should be avoided secondary to the risk of heart block and bradycardias.[4] The use of CCBs may be especially beneficial for stroke reduction and may slow the progression of atherosclerosis of the carotid arteries more than beta blockers.[14] CCBs can be used to reduce proteinuria if ACE inhibitors are poorly tolerated or in conjunction with ACE inhibitors or ARBs. ARBs, CCBs, and thiazide diuretics have been most consistent in showing cardiovascular benefits.

Second-line pharmacologic agents can be used when comorbidities affect clinical decision-making for hypertensive patients. Beta-blockers can be used as a first-line drug after myocardial infarction or in patients with stable ischemic heart disease as there is compelling evidence of clinical benefit. Metoprolol succinate or bisoprolol is preferred if patients have heart failure with a reduced ejection fraction. Loop diuretics may be used in patients with symptomatic heart failure or moderate to severe CKD, as evidenced by a GFR < 30 mL/min. Aldosterone agonist diuretics are preferred agents as an add-on therapy for patients with primary aldosteronism or resistant hypertension. Alpha 1 blockers can be considered in patients with concurrent benign prostatic hypertrophy but can cause orthostatic hypotension in the older population. Centrally acting alpha2 agonists should be reserved as a third-line drug in the event of adverse effects on the central nervous system and rebound hypertension.[4]

Considerations

Approximately 95% of cases of hypertension are multifactorial and polygenic, and we refer to this group as primary hypertension.[18] Recent genome-wide association studies (GWAS) have identified several rare secondary hypertension forms with genetic mechanisms. Although GWAS have identified > 500 genomic targets for hypertension-relevant research, most Mendelian mechanisms are responsive to medications currently in use.[19]

SUMMARY

There has been substantial progress in our understanding of hypertension through high-quality, evidence-based research. This wealth of evidence has been translated into highly effective pharmacologic and non-pharmacologic guidelines for therapy to reduce this globally significant but preventable cause of cardiovascular disease.[14]

CLINICS CARE POINTS

- The prevalence of hypertension is increasing globally despite highly effective pharmacologic and non-pharmacological therapies currently available.
- Screening for hypertension should be undertaken in all adults and the diagnosis of hypertension is based on an average of readings over multiple visits.
- Ambulatory blood pressure measurements may help to identify masked hypertension and white coat syndromes.
- A clinical evaluation is necessary during hypertensive diagnosis to assess for cardiovascular risk factors and the presence of hypertensive mediated organ damage.
- Healthy lifestyle changes are used in both the prevention and treatment of hypertension.
- Primary hypertension can be effectively treated with drugs from five categories: angiotensin-converting enzyme, angiotensin receptor blocker, calcium channel blocker (CCB) dihydropyridines, CCB non-dihydropyridines and thiazide or thiazide-type diuretics. However, other secondary agents are available if comorbidities dictate their use.
- Secondary hypertension is rare but more likely to occur in early or sudden onset disease or resistant and severe hypertension.
- Combination therapy may be more effective than monotherapy, but a single pill therapy may increase adherence.
- Blood pressure goals for persons with or without atherosclerotic cardiovascular disease of <130/80 are reasonable targets.

DISCLOSURE

No disclosures for commercial or financial conflicts of interest.

REFERENCES

1. Sternlicht H, Bakris GL. Hypertension: a companion to braunwald's heart disease. Elsevier; 2017. https://doi.org/10.1016/b978-0-323-42973-3.00033-0.
2. Polak-Iwaniuk A, Harasim-Symbor E, Gołaszewska K, et al. How hypertension affects heart metabolism. Front Physiol 2019;10. https://doi.org/10.3389/fphys.2019.00435.
3. Yoon S, Gu Q, Nwankwo T, et al. Trends in blood pressure among adults with hypertension. Hypertension 2015;65(1):54–61.
4. Whelton PK, Carey RM, Aronow WS, et al. 2017 ACC/AHA/AAPA/ABC/ACPM/AGS/APHA/ASH/ASPC/NMA/PCNA guideline for the prevention, detection,

evaluation, and management of high blood pressure in adults: a report of the American College Of Cardiology/American Heart Association task force on clinical practice guidelines. Hypertension 2018;71(6). https://doi.org/10.1161/hyp.0000000000000065.

5. Unger T, Borghi C, Charchar F, et al. 2020 international society of hypertension global hypertension practice guidelines. J Hypertens 2020;38(6):982–1004.

6. Rader F, Victor RG. The slow evolution of blood pressure monitoring. JACC: Basic Translational Sci 2017;2(6):643–5.

7. Magder S. The meaning of blood pressure. Crit Care 2018;22(1). https://doi.org/10.1186/s13054-018-2171-1.

8. Harold JG. Historical perspectives on hypertension. Cardiol Mag 2017;1–4.

9. Lloyd-Jones DM. General population risk and global cardiovascular risk. In: Bakris GL, Sorrentino MJ, editors. Hypertension. Philadelphia, PA: Elsevier; 2018. p. 1–13.

10. Hall ME, Hall JE. Pathogenesis of hypertension. In: Hypertension: a companion to braunwald's heart disease. Elsevier; 2017. p. 33–51. https://doi.org/10.1016/b978-0-323-42973-3.00005-6.

11. Harrison D. Inflammation and immunity in hypertension. In: Bernstein K, editor. Hypertension. 3rd edition. Philadelphia: Elsevier; 2018. p. 60.

12. Johnson RJ, Lanaspa MA, Gabriela Sánchez-Lozada L, et al. The discovery of hypertension: evolving views on the role of the kidneys, and current hot topics. Am J Physiology-Renal Physiol 2015;308(3):F167–78.

13. Loperena R, Harrison DG. Oxidative stress and hypertensive diseases. Med Clin North Am 2017;101(1):169–93.

14. Williams B, Mancia G, Spiering W, et al. 2018 ESC/ESH guidelines for the management of arterial hypertension. J Hypertens 2018;36(10):1953–2041.

15. Carey RM, Muntner P, Bosworth HB, et al. Prevention and control of hypertension. J Am Coll Cardiol 2018;72(11):1278–93.

16. National Heart, Lung, and Blood Institute & National Heart, Lung, and Blood Institute. Your guide to lowering your blood pressure with DASH. 1st edition. Betheda, MD: National Heart, Lung, and Blood Institute; 2006.

17. Lopes J, Fonseca M, Torres-Costoso A, et al. Low- and moderate-intensity aerobic exercise acutely reduce blood pressure in adults with high-normal/grade I hypertension. J Clin Hypertens 2020;22(9):1732–6.

18. Kolifarhood G, Daneshpour M, Hadaegh F, et al. Heritability of blood pressure traits in diverse populations: a systematic review and meta-analysis. J Hum Hypertens 2019;33(11):775–85.

19. Luft FC. Molecular genetics of human hypertension. Curr Opin Cardiol 2020;35(3):249–57.

Cardiorenal Syndromes
Evaluation and Management

Leanne H. Fowler, DNP, MBA, AGACNP-BC, CNE*,
Cathy McAtee, DNP, ACNP-BC, CNE

KEYWORDS

- Cardiorenal syndrome • Acute heart failure • Chronic heart failure
- Cardiorenal syndrome biomarkers • Acute kidney injury • Chronic kidney disease

KEY POINTS

- Cardiorenal syndromes (CRS) are not common but have detrimental patient outcomes contributing to an increased burden of cardiac and kidney disease if not death.
- There are 5 types of cardiorenal syndrome classifications.
- A cycle of organ injuries occur through mechanisms of overactivation of neurohormonal and inflammatory mechanisms, circulation of free radicals, and oxidative stress that results in heart and kidney tissue fibrosis and CRS.
- Diagnosing CRS requires identification of clinical findings and diagnostic tests.
- The use of novel biomarkers aid in the evaluation and management of patients with CRS.

CARDIORENAL SYNDROME: DIAGNOSIS AND MANAGEMENT
Introduction

Cardiorenal syndrome (CRS) is a physiological disorder involving heart failure exacerbation subsequently causing renal failure or vice versa.[1] The syndrome is defined as disorders of the heart and kidneys where acute or chronic dysfunction of one organ induces acute or chronic dysfunction of the other.[2] The burden of disease is high for heart failure and kidney failure independently, thereby making CRS often associated with critical illness, high risk for overall morbidity and mortality, poor patient outcomes overall, and poor quality of life.[3,4] Furthermore, CRS can be accelerated and/or complicated by occurring in patients with comorbidities of chronic cardiovascular disease (CVD; especially atrial fibrillation and peripheral arterial disease) and chronic diabetes mellitus (DM).[1] All nurses should recognize CRS and consider the patient's severity of illness in their clinical reasoning for the evaluation and management of this patient population across all settings.

Louisiana State University Health New Orleans School of Nursing, 1900 Gravier Street, New Orleans, LA 70112, USA
* Corresponding author.
E-mail address: lfowle@lsuhsc.edu

Crit Care Nurs Clin N Am 34 (2022) 383–393
https://doi.org/10.1016/j.cnc.2022.08.001
ccnursing.theclinics.com

Background

There are 5 classifications of CRS described in **Table 1**.[5] The epidemiology of each subtype has not been clearly studied in the United States or internationally.[6] However, the prevalence of certain types is well known. For example, CRS is highest among hospitalized patients with acute or progressive heart failure who already have underlying kidney disease.[7] Additionally, approximately 16% of all hospitalized patients diagnosed with acute kidney injury (AKI) will develop CRS type 1[8]; and recovery of kidney function when CRS develops is not common.[3] Almost half of all heart failure cases involve some degree of chronic kidney disease (CKD) and similarly, patients living with CKD or end-stage kidney disease (ESKD) also live with some degree of CVD. When diagnosed with CRS, mortality rates are highest among patients with declining cardiovascular disease and severe CKD or those requiring dialysis.[4,7,9] The diagnosis of CRS offers the patient a poor prognosis.[4,9]

Disease pathology

The heart and kidneys have a symbiotic relationship where one system directly effects and depends on the other system, and both are highly dependent on the complex interplay of fluid volume supporting each organ's function. As each organ becomes injured, the cascade of pathological processes produces a cycle of injuries between the 2 organs and ultimately, the development of CRS. The exact pathologic mechanisms of CRS are unclear but regardless of the mechanisms of injury to the heart and/or kidneys, the pathological processes involved include increased inflammation and circulation of free radicals causing endothelial cell injury, oxidative stress, and fibrosis of the architectural structure of the heart and/or kidneys.[10–12] Drug toxicities can also contribute to kidney injury when combined with the other pathophysiologic processes causing CRS. The cycle of acute organ injuries occurs from increased levels of inflammatory biomarkers, oxidative stress, and endothelial dysfunction and leads to the fibrotic remodeling of cardiac and/or renal tissue.[11,12]

The pathologic condition of type 1 and type 2 CRS begins with acute or chronic cardiac failure where decreased cardiac output and increased blood pressures activate the renin-angiotensin-aldosterone system and overall reduced perfusion to the kidneys resulting in acute or worsened CKD. The pathologic condition of type 3 and type 4 CRS begins with acute or chronic renal failure evidenced by uremia, electrolyte disorders, and fluid volume overload leading to arrythmias, impaired tissue perfusion, and decline in cardiac function.[11]

The pathologic mechanisms involved in type 5 CRS begins with an acute systemic inflammatory response to severe illness of one or more organs (eg, sepsis, acute severe pancreatitis, acute severe pneumonia). The same mechanisms of injury from inflammation, oxidative stress, free radicals, and endothelial can cause new or compounding injury to the heart and kidneys.[11] Without improvement of the systemic illness, the injuries to the heart and kidneys continue and can lead to CRS. Patients with underlying chronic heart and kidney disease have a higher risk for developing type 5 CRS than those without both comorbidities.[12]

Patient Evaluation

A prudent and careful patient interview can inform the nurse of the symptoms of both heart and renal failure. Building on the history, the physical examination findings should focus on the signs patients may not know how to articulate during the encounter. Furthermore, patients may not know the significance of the signs and symptoms of CRS. Therefore, the nurse should complete a comprehensive history and physical examination unless the patient is hemodynamically unstable. In the event

Table 1
Classifications of cardiorenal syndromes[3,4]

Classification Type	Etiologies	Clinical Characteristics	Pathophysiology Mechanism(s)
Type 1—Acute CRS	Acute ischemic heart disease, Cardiogenic shock, ADHF	ADHF causing AKI	Sympathetic hyperactivity Constriction of afferent and efferent arterioles ↓renal perfusion RAAS activation ↑sodium and water retention Venous congestion ↓renal perfusion pressure gradient
Type 2—Chronic CRS	Chronic heart failure	Chronic cardiac dysfunction leading to progressive CKD	↓renal plasma flow, elevated efferent arteriolar resistance
Type 3—Acute renocardiac syndrome	AKI, uremia, hyperkalemia, Volume overload causing pulmonary edema	AKI leading to acute cardiac dysfunction	Cardiac dysfunction caused by volume overload from AKI, inflammatory cascade
Type 4—Chronic renocardiac syndrome	CKD-associated cardiomyopathy	CKD leading to progressive chronic cardiac dysfunction	Remodeling of the myocardium (CKD-associated cardiomyopathy)
Type 5—Secondary CRS	DM, sepsis, amyloidosis, cirrhosis	Acute or progressive chronic systemic disorder leading to cardiac and renal dysfunction	↓ renal blood flow in sepsis connective tissue diseases diabetes

Abbreviations: ADHF, Acute decompensating heart failure; RAAS, renin-angiotensin-aldosterone system.

the patient is hemodynamically unstable, when stabilized, the nurse should obtain a comprehensive history and examination from the patient and or family. Advanced practice nurses should initially develop a broad differential diagnoses and then use the clinical findings and diagnostic tests to define the diagnosis.

Patient history

Patients presenting with CRS can report symptoms related to the primary disease process—cardiac, renal, or systemic. However, patients may also have characteristics indicating the progression of CRS along a confluent pathologic continuum. A careful history can help to identify the initial insult; however, due to the overlapping nature of cardiac and renal pathologic conditions, the true insult instigating the CRS cascade could be difficult to differentiate.[13] To improve early recognition of CRS, the nurse should apply the patient's symptoms to the characteristic findings of the CRS classifications (**Table 2**).[14] Systemic symptoms such as fever, fatigue, unintentional weight loss, or weight gain can make differentiating CRS classifications more difficult. Additionally, weight trends and a careful history of fluid losses may be helpful in discriminating the CRS causes related to fluid volume changes.

Past medical history. The patient's medical history can help nurses to distinguish which system was injured first and, possibly, the CRS classification. For instance, a past medical history of CVD with known ejection fraction of 35%, insulin-dependent diabetes mellitus (IDDM), and CKD with known normal baseline kidney function could offer the nurse clues to which organ led to CRS. Reviewing the home medications can also be helpful clues for a prior history of cardiac, renal, or another organ dysfunction and current use of potentially nephrotoxic medications or herbal supplements.

Social history. Patients living with alcohol use disorder are at risk for developing dilated cardiomyopathy, cirrhosis of the liver, and kidney injury/disease, which are all risk factors for CRS. Similarly, tobacco use disorder or illicit drug abuse increases the patient's risk for CVD generally and impaired heart and/or kidney function. Collecting a thorough sexual history may also be helpful in identifying the patient's risk factors for infectious diseases such as viral hepatitis that could potentially progress to liver dysfunction or failure and kidney disease.

Physical examination

Using clues obtained from the comprehensive patient history, a comprehensive physical examination should be performed to carefully evaluate each body system. Discerning signs indicative of acute or chronic cardiac, renal, or other organ system failure is necessary to help differentiate CRS classifications. Examination findings aligned to CRS classifications and types are noted in **Table 2**.[3,15]

Differential diagnoses

Advanced practice nurses' scope of practice includes developing differential diagnoses before initiating a prioritized management plan. The differential diagnoses for CRS can be difficult to differentiate but should include problems associated with acute or chronic heart failure, renal failure, fluid volume overload or volume deficit, nephrotoxicity, or type 5 CRS (**Box 1**). Developing broad differential diagnoses initially from clinical findings and then narrowing them down with diagnostic tests will help nurses identify or have high suspicion for CRS.

Diagnostic testing

Diagnostic serum, urine, and radiographic tests help to define organ failure and classify CRS. Evaluating the biomarkers, inflammatory markers, and overall

Table 2
Clinical findings and treatments for cardiorenal syndromes[3,15]

Cardiorenal Syndrome Classification	Patient Symptoms	Physical Examination	Treatment
Type 1—Acute CRS	Fatigue, generalized weakness, acute and exertional dyspnea, orthopnea, paroxysmal nocturnal dyspnea , syncope, chest pain, palpitations, swelling	Weight gain, Jugular vein distention (JVD), labored respirations, Bibasilar crackles, S3 gallop, dependent central and/or peripheral edema, disorientation to encephalopathy, asterixis	Diuresis with loop and thiazide type diuretics, acetazolamide, ultrafiltration inotropes for resistant congestion
Type 2—Chronic CRS	Any of the above described as progressive onset	Any of the above and pruritis, ascites	Treat underlying HF cardiac resynchronization therapy
Type 3—Acute renocardiac syndrome	Any of the above and arrythmias, muscle cramps	Any of the above findings with renal symptoms occurring first	Treat underlying AKI
Type 4—Chronic renocardiac syndrome	Any of those above	Any of the above findings with progressive renal symptoms occurring first	RAAS inhibitors MRAs
Type 5—Secondary CRS	Any of the above and fever, altered mental status, easy bleeding and bruising, neuropathic pain and/or paresthesia	Any of the above symptoms and hepatomegaly, exanthem, sensory deficits	Treat sepsis or underlying systemic disease

Box 1
Differential diagnoses for cardiorenal syndrome

Heart Failure
    Acute myocardial infarction
    Cardiomyopathy
    Overdose
    Amyloidosis
    Infectious myocarditis or pericarditis
    Inflammatory myocarditis or pericarditis

Renal Failure
    Acute kidney injury
        Infectious nephritis
    Chronic kidney disease
        Glomerulonephritis
        Glomerulosclerosis
        Lupus nephritis
        Renal artery stenosis
    Nephrotoxicity

Hypervolemia
    Psychogenic water intoxication
    Renal Failure

Hypovolemia
    Vomiting and/or diarrhea
        Infectious or inflammatory enteritis
    Malnutrition

Shock syndrome
    Sepsis
    Cardiogenic
    Hypovolemic/hemorrhagic
    Anaphylactic
    Neurogenic

neurohormonal cross talk between the heart and kidneys during acute injury is necessary for the diagnosis of CRS.[4] A complete blood count and comprehensive metabolic panel as general medical screening tests for blood loss, indications of infection or inflammation, electrolyte imbalances, and organ dysfunction should also be ordered.

Hemodynamic measurements of intracardiac pressures can be obtained from pulmonary artery catheters or noninvasive devices to evaluate cardiac function. The measures of cardiac output, central venous pressure, pulmonary artery, and occlusive pressures can help measure and trend cardiac function. There is an 88% correlation between an elevated pulmonary artery occlusive pressure and central venous pressure in patients with advanced heart failure.[15]

Biomarkers. The use of novel biomarkers along with traditional diagnostic studies adds a new dimension to the evaluation of organ damage and injury and can also serve as a guide to therapeutic strategies for CRS. The biomarker cystatin C (CysC) when combined with NT-proBNP and troponin T is a powerful predictor of rehospitalization and both short-term and long-term morbidity in patients with advanced heart failure (AHF).[4] However, the nurse should consider that NT-proBNP and troponin T can be falsely elevated secondary to reduced renal clearance.[16] Albuminuria has a strong correlation with readmission, cardiovascular death, and all-cause mortality in heart failure patients across multiple major HF trials.[4] Fractional excretion of urine sodium (FeNa) less than 1% and urea less than 35 mg/dL indicate prerenal AKI, along with biomarkers of cell-cycle arrest such as urine insulin-like growth factor-binding 7 (IGFBP7) and tissue inhibitor of metalloproteinase 2 (TIMP-2), can assist the clinician in identifying AHF patients that are most at risk for progressing into a CRS cascade.[15] These biomarkers of tubular integrity can help identify those at risk for acute renal failure or CRS and can help distinguish AKI from prerenal azotemia.[17]

Diagnostic imaging. Ultrasound imaging of the heart, kidneys, and renal blood flow can be used to help diagnose CRS and guide treatment therapies.[18] For instance, an ultrasound with Doppler evaluation of the renal vessels is used to evaluate the patient for vascular causes of renal failure but can also help to guide diuretic therapy and reduce the incidence of overdiuresis.[19] Echocardiography is the gold standard for to evaluate cardiac function, estimate filling pressures, calculate the ejection fraction, and evaluate systolic and diastolic cardiac function.[16]

Patient Management

The management of CRS is as complex as the disease process. Additionally, each patient may have nuanced presentations based on the type of CRS and their personal underlying comorbidities. Timely identification and evidence-based management strategies can help to improve patient outcomes.

Pharmacotherapies

Loop diuretics are the first-line therapy for hypervolemia; other diuretics can be used as adjunctive therapy if diuresis is suboptimal.[15] There is no significant difference in outcomes whether continuous infusions or bolus doses of loop diuretics are used. A diuretic challenge of 1.0 to 1.5 mg/kg of IV furosemide can predict the risk of progressive AKI, the need for renal replacement therapy (RRT), and poorer outcomes if urine output is less than 200 cc within 2 hours after dosing.[7] Diuretic resistance is common in the renal patient due to uremic toxins competing with diuretics for organic anion transporters and secretion in the proximal convoluted tubule. It is estimated that only 10% to 20% of the loop diuretic is secreted into the proximal tubule in uremic patients with creatine clearance less than 15 mL/min. By combining a loop with a thiazide-like diuretic such as metolazone, sodium reabsorption in the proximal tubule is prevented thereby augmenting diuresis and improving congestive symptoms.[15] However, this is accompanied by an increased risk of electrolyte derangements.[7] All decongestive pharmacological therapies are aimed at restoring the perfusion gradient across the glomerular capillary bed and improving glomerular filtration rate (GFR), despite seemingly increased creatine levels from the correction of hypervolemia.[3,13] Serum creatinine should not be used to guide diuretic therapy in the setting of acute decompensated heart failure (ADHF) because an increase in serum creatinine is to be expected in 33% of cases.[13,14] A reasonable goal of therapy is monitoring urine output to ensure a negative fluid balance of 2 to 3 L in the first 24 hours of admission in patients with severe congestion.[15] Holding or decreasing diuretic dosages in ADHF based on serum creatinine levels can have detrimental effects on patient outcomes such as increased readmission rates and higher mortality.[13]

Renin-angiotensin-aldosterone system (RAAS) inhibiting drugs such as angiotensin-converting enzyme (ACE) inhibitors and angiotensin receptor blockers have been a mainstay of therapy for both heart failure and CKD during the past 2 decades. These drugs are universally prescribed to all patients with heart failure with reduced ejection fraction (HFrEF) and/or CKD for their well-known cardiorenal protective mechanism secondary to RAAS inhibition.[20] Although it is reasonable to continue this therapy in the presence of mild AKI, therapy should be withheld during episodes of severe AKI and resumed during the recovery phase of AKI.[7,16] Although there is a decrease in estimated GFR related to the initiation of RAAS inhibitors, long-term cardiovascular outcomes are improved in the HFrEF population. A post hoc analysis of the Prospective Comparison of ARNI with ACEI to Determine Impact on Global Mortality and Morbidity (PARADIGM)-Heart Failure (HF) trial showed additional cardiovascular and renal benefits from sacubitril/neprilysin therapy compared with those from ACE inhibitors alone. Renal benefits were realized despite a slight increase in the urinary albumin/creatinine ratio, which stabilized with continued sacubitril/neprilysin use.[21]

RAAS inhibition does not provide complete suppression of sympathetic activation and the phenomenon of aldosterone escape can occur with long-term ACE inhibitor/angiotensin receptor blocker (ARB) therapy. Adding a mineralocorticoid receptor agonist (MRA) to an ACE inhibitor/ARB can provide additional RAAS suppression and reduce serum aldosterone as well as sodium and water retention. Research indicates that adjunctive MRAs use in HF reduces CV events and mortality in patients with and without CKD, although the data on CKD 4 and 5 are extremely limited.[4,22]

Inotropic therapy with dobutamine or milrinone can be used for hemodynamic support during cardiogenic shock states to maintain adequate organ perfusion. Its use in acute cardiorenal syndrome may be of some benefit, especially when resistance to diuretic therapy exists. Therapeutic benefits include increasing cardiac output, right ventricular output, and renal perfusion, which would in turn decrease systemic congestion.[15] Although inotropes are effective in this subgroup of CRS with hypotension, the practice of routine use of inotropes for CRS should be avoided.[7]

Numerous trials have shown that sodium-glucose cotransporter 2 inhibitors (SGLT2i) have been shown in numerous trials to provide significant cardiovascular benefits, with 30% to 40% reduction in hospitalizations for heart failure in patients with CKD. The primary mechanism of preload reduction is by preventing glucose and sodium reabsorption in the proximal tubule and promoting glycosuria and natriuresis.[23] SGLT2i and glucagon-like peptide agonists (GLP) provide cardiorenal protection in addition to their glucose-lowering properties. Recent research, such as the Dapagliflozin and Prevention of Adverse-outcomes in Heart Failure (DAPA-HF) study, has found that dapagliflozin may be of clinical benefit to HFrEF management in the absence of type 2 diabetes mellitus (T2DM) diagnosis.[24]

Nonpharmacological therapies

Management strategies for patients with advanced heart failure should include a multidisciplinary approach with follow-up in a dedicated heart failure center until their condition has stabilized.[15] Nephrology consultation and follow-up has been shown to be an effective strategy to reduce all-cause mortality following an AKI event.[16]

Ultrafiltration is a second line therapy that is capable of removing iso-osmolar fluid at a steady and predictable rate that can be individualized based on clinical parameters. This therapy is reserved for patients who are resistant to diuretic therapies at their maximum dose, are severely overloaded with fluid, acidotic, and unresponsive to medical management.[15,16] Continuous renal replacement therapies can be used in the hemodynamically unstable patient to facilitate improvement of acid–base disturbances. Studies that compare ultrafiltration alone to diuretic therapies do not show a benefit to ultrafiltration that may cause volume depletion in a malnourished patient who has low oncotic pressure and slow plasma refill.[15]

Cardiac resynchronization. Biventricular pacing and resynchronization therapy has been found to improve both heart failure and CRS outcomes such as reduced hospitalizations and improved quality of life.[4] Use of this device has reduced the need for transplantation or left ventricular assist devices and prevented death by way of increasing cardiac output and mean arterial pressure and reducing venous congestion and central venous pressure (CVP).[11]

Left ventricular assist device. In selective patients with refractory heart failure long-term mechanical circulatory support (MCS) can be used as a bridge to transplant in patients with mild-to-moderate CKD and cases of advanced CKD, if the patient is a good candidate for heart and kidney transplant (KT). There is generally an immediate improvement seen in renal functions that dissipates over time for unknown reasons, so advanced CKD is a relative contraindication to MCS therapy if transplant is unlikely.[25]

Transplantation. To underscore the convergent relationship between the heart and the kidneys, it has been observed that postoperative EF improved to a mean of 52% in post KT patients with HFrEF and a mean EF of 32%. Uremic cardiomyopathy changes were noted to reverse in selected case studies. This raises the question of the appropriateness of HFrEF as a contraindication for KT and the need to extend dialysis while waiting for heart transplant and KT because pretransplant dialysis duration is inversely related to EF improvement after KT.[26]

DISCUSSION

The development of CRS is most common among patients with chronic heart and/or kidney disease. However, the cycle of acute injuries between the heart and kidneys or from a systemic illness can progress to CRS. The development of CRS offers patients a poor prognosis. Nurses should understand and apply the pathological processes of CRS to aid in its early identification and treatment. Future nursing research is needed to study if nurse-driven protocols improve patient outcomes.

CLINICS CARE POINTS

- Evaluate patients at risk for heart-kidney interactions during acute illness.
- Evaluate risk factors of patients with chronic illness who are at risk for CRS during acute illness (e.g. HF, CKD or ESKD, DM, kidney transplant recipients).
- Loop diuretics, ACE-Is or ARBs, and MRAs are routine pharmacotherapies when not contraindicated for acute renal toxicity.
- The routine use of inotropic therapy should be avoided in patients with CRS.
- Heart or kidney transplantation can improve either organ's function.
- Palliative care may have a role in the management of patients with CRS.

DISCLOSURE

The authors have no financial disclosures or other conflicts of interest.

REFERENCES

1. Goldstein J, Dieter RS, Bansal V, et al. Arterial-renal syndrome in patients with ESRD, a new disease paradigm. Clin Appl Thromb Hemost 2022;28:1–6.

2. Ronco C, McCullough P, Anker SD, et al. Cardio-renal syndromes: report from the consensus conference of the acute dialysis quality initiative. Eur Heart J 2009;31: 703–11.
3. Raina R, Nair N, Chakraborty R, et al. An update on the pathophysiology and treatment of cardiorenal syndrome. Cardiol Res 2020;11:76–88.
4. Rangaswami J, Bhalla V, Blair JE, et al. Cardiorenal syndrome: classification, pathophysiology, diagnosis, and treatment strategies: a scientific statement from the american heart association. Circulation 2019;139(16). https://doi.org/10.1161/cir.0000000000000664.
5. Buliga-Finis ON, Ouatu A, Badescu MC, et al. Beyond the cardiorenal syndrome: pathophysiological approaches and biomarkers for renal and cardiac crosstalk. Diagnostics 2022;12:1–17.
6. Uduman J. Epidemiology of cardiorenal syndrome. Adv Chronic Kidney Dis 2018; 25(5):391–9.
7. Jentzer JC, Bihorac A, Brusca SB, et al. Contemporary management of severe acute kidney injury and refractory cardiorenal syndrome. J Am Coll Cardiol 2020;76(9):1084–101.
8. Seckinger D, Ritter O, Patschan D. Risk factors and outcome variables of cardiorenal syndrome type 1 from the nephrologist's perspective. Int Urol Nephrol 2022;54:1591–601.
9. McCullough PA, Amin A, Pantalone KM, et al. Cardiorenal Nexus: a review with focus on combined chronic heart and kidney failure, and insights from recent clinical trials. J Am Heart Assoc 2022;11(11):1–9.
10. Yeh JN, Yue Y, Chu YC, et al. J Biomed Pharmacother 2021;144:1–20.
11. Verma D, Firoz A, Garlapati S, et al. Emerging treatments of cardiorenal syndrome: an update on pathophysiology and management. Cureus 2021. https://doi.org/10.7759/cureus.17240.
12. Delgado-Valero B, Cachofeiro V, Martinez-Martinez E. Fibrosis, the bad actor in cardiorenal syndromes: mechanisms involved. Cells 2021;10(7):1824.
13. Kumar U, Wettersten N, Garimella PS. Cardiorenal syndrome. Cardiol Clin 2019; 201937(3):251–65.
14. Hatamizadeh P. Cardiorenal syndrome. Cardiol Clin 2021;39(3):455–69.
15. Thind GS, Loehrke M, Wilt JL. Acute cardiorenal syndrome: mechanisms and clinical implications. Cleve Clin J Med 2018;85(3):231–9.
16. Legrand M, Rossignol P. Cardiovascular consequences of acute kidney injury. N Engl J Med 2020;382(23):2238–47.
17. Ataci A, Cakmak R, Yuruyen G, et al. Type I cardiorenal syndrome in patients with acutely decompensated heart failure: the importance of new renal biomarkers. Eur Rev Med Pharmacol Sci 2018;11:3534–43.
18. Ricci Z, Romagnoli S, Ronco C. Cardiorenal syndrome. Crit Care Clin 2021;37(2): 335–47.
19. Çakal B, Özcan Ö, Omaygenç M, et al. Value of renal vascular Doppler sonography in cardiorenal syndrome type 1. J Ultrasound Med 2020;40(2):321–30.
20. Rossignol P. A step forward toward a new treatment paradigm in the cardiorenal continuum. JACC: Heart Fail 2021;9(11):821–3.
21. Damman K, Gori M, Claggett B, et al. Renal effects and associated outcomes during angiotensin-neprilysin inhibition in heart failure. JACC: Heart Fail 2018; 6(6):489–98.
22. Yancy CW, Jessup M, Bozkurt B, et al. 2017 ACC/AHA/HFSA focused update of the 2013 ACCF/AHA guideline for the management of heart failure: a report of the american college of cardiology/american heart association task force on clinical

practice guidelines and the heart failure society of America. Circulation 2017; 136(6). https://doi.org/10.1161/cir.0000000000000509.

23. Dou L, Burtey S. Reversing endothelial dysfunction with empagliflozin to improve cardiomyocyte function in cardiorenal syndrome. Kidney Int 2021;99(5):1062–4.

24. Kalra S, Sahay M, Ghosh S, et al. Cardiorenal syndrome in type 2 diabetes mellitus- Rational use of sodium-glucose cotransporter-2 inhibitors. Eur Endocrinol 2020;2:113–21.

25. Cowger JA, Radjef R. Advanced heart failure therapies and cardiorenal syndrome. Adv Chronic Kidney Dis 2018;25(5):443–53.

26. Josephson CB, Delgado D, Schiff J, et al. The effectiveness of renal transplantation as a treatment for recurrent uremic cardiomyopathy. Can J Cardiol 2008; 24(4):315–7.

Complications in Patients with Chronic Kidney Disease

Kevin M. Lowe, MSN, APRN, ACNP-BC, CNN-NP[a],*,
Jan Buenacosa Cruz, MSN, MPH, APRN, NP-C, CNN-NP[b],
Katerina M. Jones, DNP, APRN, ANP-C, CNN-NP[a,1]

KEYWORDS

- Chronic kidney disease (CKD) • Complications • Anemia
- Bone–mineral metabolism • Hypertension • Hyperkalemia • Metabolic acidosis
- Cardiovascular disease

KEY POINTS

- Chronic kidney disease (CKD) affects millions of people worldwide and contributes to millions of deaths yearly, with cardiovascular disease as the leading cause of death.
- CKD is progressive and associated with several clinical complications as kidney function declines; these include cardiovascular disease, dyslipidemia, hypertension, fluid overload, electrolyte abnormalities, acid–base abnormalities, anemia, mineral–bone disorders.
- CKD management is aimed at slowing disease progression after diagnosis, detection of CKD complications, and identification of potentially reversible etiologies.

INTRODUCTION

Chronic kidney disease (CKD) is estimated to affect between 8 and 16% of the world's population and contributes to as many as 1.2 million deaths per year, with cardiovascular disease remaining the leading cause of death in these individuals.[1,2] The United States Renal Data System 2021 annual data reports nearly 15% of the US population has CKD.[3] CKD is defined as having an estimated glomerular filtration rate (eGFR) of less than 60 mL/min per 1.73 m,[2] urine albumin excretion of at least 30 mg/24 h, or markers of kidney damage that include hematuria or structural abnormalities that is present for at least three months.[1,2,4] CKD in the United States is most commonly associated with diabetes and hypertension. Early screening and detection of CKD is key in preventing negative associated clinical outcomes, with most patients presenting asymptomatically.[1] CKD is often progressive and associated with several clinical complications as kidney function deteriorates.

CKD management is aimed at slowing disease progression after diagnosis, detection of CKD complications, and identification of potentially reversible etiologies.

[a] Metrolina Nephrology Associates, Charlotte, NC, USA; [b] Rocky Mountain Regional VA Medical Center, 1700 N. Wheeling St, Aurora, CO 80045, USA
[1] Present address: 2544 Court Dr. Suite F, Gastonia, NC 28054.
* Corresponding author. 7903 Providence Rd. Suite 110, Charlotte, NC 28277.
E-mail address: KevinLoweNP@gmail.com

Crit Care Nurs Clin N Am 34 (2022) 395–407
https://doi.org/10.1016/j.cnc.2022.07.005
ccnursing.theclinics.com
0899-5885/22/© 2022 Elsevier Inc. All rights reserved.

Associated complications include hypertension, fluid overload, electrolyte abnormalities, acid–base abnormalities, anemia, mineral–bone disease disorder and cardiovascular disease.[5] Once CKD progresses to end-stage kidney disease (ESKD), symptoms of uremia may develop. Health care providers should be aware of complications associated with CKD, as sequelae of these complications often contribute to disease progression necessitating the use of renal replacement therapy in addition to increased patient morbidity and mortality.

DISCUSSION
Definition and Staging of Chronic Kidney Disease

The initial 2002 National Kidney Foundation–Kidney Disease Outcomes Quality Initiative guidelines for the evaluation, classification, and stratification of CKD had a significant impact on the diagnosis and management of individuals with CKD.[6] However, nephrologists recognized the need to update this initiative as new information became available. In particular, albuminuria was identified as an independent predictor of negative clinical outcomes and was incorporated into the 2012 updated KDIGO Clinical Practice Guideline for the Evaluation and Management of CKD.[6] The latest KDIGO (Kidney Disease: Improving Global Outcomes) publication defines CKD as abnormalities of kidney structure or function, present for >3 months, with implications for health.[4] CKD is further classified based on etiology, GFR category, and the extent of albuminuria present.[4] The KDIGO heat map (**Fig. 1**) is commonly used to visualize the relationship between eGFR and albuminuria and associated risk of CKD progression.

KDIGO guidelines recommend the use of a GFR estimating equation for accurate assessment of kidney function. All existing equations for eGFR include variables, which account for muscle mass, including age, gender, height, weight, and race.[7] The use of race in eGFR has limitations, with self-reported race correlating imperfectly with genomic ancestry and thus with muscle mass. There has been increased attention recently toward obtaining more accurate measures of eGFR and removing the race variable.[7] In a study by Inker and colleagues, new eGFR equations were used which incorporate both serum creatinine and cystatin C, and further omit race as a modifier in calculating eGFR. This has been shown to be more accurate, and led to smaller differences between Black participants and non-Black participants when compared to equations without race with either creatinine or cystatin C alone. Thus, the NKF-ASN task force in 2021 presented their recommendations on reassessing the inclusion of race in diagnosing kidney disease.[8] These include (1) implementation of the CKD-EPI creatinine equation refit without the race variable in all laboratories in the United States; (2) facilitate the increased, routine, and timely use of cystatin C measures and other validated equations refitted without a race variable to confirm estimated GFR in adults at risk for or with known kidney disease; and (3) continued research and funding on GFR estimation with new endogenous filtration markers and other interventions to eliminate race and ethnic disparities.

Once diagnosed, CKD is staged based on GFR and albuminuria. There are six stages of GFR and three stages of albuminuria. **Table 1** outlines the stages of GFR and albuminuria.

COMPLICATIONS OF CHRONIC KIDNEY DISEASE
Cardiovascular Disease and Dyslipidemia

Cardiovascular disease is the leading cause of death in patients with CKD, with incidence and mortality increasing as CKD advances and eGFR declines.[2,9,10] Traditional risk factors, such as hypertension, insulin resistance/diabetes, obesity, dyslipidemia,

				Persistent albuminuria categories Description and range		
				A1	A2	A3
Prognosis of CKD by GFR and Albuminuria Categories: KDIGO 2012				Normal to mildly increased	Moderately increased	Severely increased
				<30 mg/g <3 mg/mmol	30-300 mg/g 3-30 mg/mmol	>300 mg/g >30 mg/mmol
GFR categories (ml/min/ 1.73 m²) Description and range	G1	Normal or high	≥90			
	G2	Mildly decreased	60–89			
	G3a	Mildly to moderately decreased	45–59			
	G3b	Moderately to severely decreased	30–44			
	G4	Severely decreased	15–29			
	G5	Kidney failure	<15			

Green: low risk (if no other markers of kidney disease, no CKD); Yellow: moderately increased risk; Orange: high risk; Red, very high risk.

Fig. 1. Prognosis of CKD by GFR and albuminuria category. (*From* Kidney Disease: Improving Global Outcomes (KDIGO) Work Group. KDIGO 2012 clinical practice guideline for the evaluation and management of chronic kidney disease. Kidney International. 2013;3:1-150.)

smoking, and sedentary lifestyle, predispose patients with CKD to cardiovascular disease at earlier stages of CKD due to their effects on kidney vasculature.[2,11] Lower eGFR and higher levels of albuminuria also contribute to an increased risk of cardiovascular events in patients with CKD.[2] Nontraditional risk factors for the development of cardiovascular disease in CKD include vascular calcification, systemic inflammatory processes, anemia, CKD-related bone–mineral disorder abnormalities, increased extracellular fluid volume, malnutrition, and endothelial dysfunction.[11–13]

Table 1
Staging of estimated glomerular filtration rate and albuminuria

Stage of GFR	Stages of Albuminuria
G1 = GFR ≥ 90 mL/min/1.73 m²	A1=<30 mg/g
G2 = GFR 60–89 mL/min/1.73 m²	A2 = 30–300 mg/g
G3a = GFR 45–59 mL/min/1.73 m²	A3= > 300 mg/g
G3b = GFR 30–44 mL/min/1.73 m²	
G4 = GFR 15–29 mL/min/1.73 m²	
G5 = GFR < 15 mL/min/1.73 m²	

Source: Chen, Knicely & Grams.[1]

Cardiovascular calcifications within central arterial vessels lead to increased cardiac afterload and ultimately heart failure, whereas calcifications of cardiac valves lead to valvular stenosis, namely aortic valve stenosis in this population.[11] Left ventricular hypertrophy (LVH) is present in approximately one-third of patients with CKD and its incidence increases to 70% to 80% by the time a patient progresses to ESKD.[11]

The presentation of cardiovascular disease in patients with CKD is often atypical. Patients with CKD are more likely to present with an acute myocardial infarction (AMI) versus stable angina. They are less likely to report typical AMI symptomology (chest, arm, shoulder, neck pain) compared with patients with preserved renal function; however, patients with CKD are more likely to present with dyspnea.[10] Patients with CKD with coronary artery disease (CAD) have a higher incidence of presenting with a non-ST-segment elevation myocardial infarction versus an ST-segment elevation myocardial infarction.[10] LVH and electrolyte abnormalities are associated with the suspected development of cardiac arrhythmias and increase the likelihood of sudden cardiac death, particularly in patients with CKD whose renal function has progressed to end-stage.[10] Screening for asymptomatic CAD is often not recommended in patients with CKD; however, this has been justified in protocols for prescreening potential renal transplant candidates.[10,13]

Prevention and treatment are often aimed at lifestyle modifications (increased physical activity, smoking cessation, etc.) as well as dyslipidemia management, diabetic A1c control, protection against albuminuria with the use of angiotensin-converting enzyme inhibitors (ACEi)/ angiotensin II receptor blockers (ARB) agents, strict blood pressure target goals, and use of sodium–glucose co-transporter 2 inhibitors. KDIGO recommends statin therapy in patients with early-stage CKD over the age of 50 years, as well as use for individuals under the age of 50 years who have ongoing risk factors.[13] There is limited evidence to support initiation of statin therapy for dialysis-dependent patients with ESKD; however, those treated with statin therapy in non-dialysis-dependent CKD should continue therapy. Sodium-glucose cotransporter 2 (SLGT2) inhibitors have been shown to have both renal and cardiac protection.[13]

Hypertension/Fluid Overload

Hypertension is one of the most common contributing factors of CKD with prevalence ranging anywhere from 60% to 90%.[14] The development of hypertension in CKD is related to total volume overload, sodium retention, sympathetic system overactivity, endothelial dysfunction, increased activity of the renin-angiotensin-aldosterone system (RAAS) and medication noncompliance.[14] While CKD causes hypertension, hypertension causes CKD and its progression; thus, the diagnosis and treatment of hypertension is paramount to the management and slowing of CKD progression. The 2021 American Heart Association/American College of Cardiology identifies normal blood pressure as <120/<80 mm Hg. Elevated blood pressure is defined as 120–129/<80 mm Hg. Stage I hypertension is defined as 130–139/80–89 mm Hg. Stage II hypertension is a reading $\geq 140/\geq 9$[15] The 2021 KDIGO guidelines now recommend a target systolic blood pressure goal of <120 mm Hg for CKD patients with diagnosed hypertension, with or without diabetes, as tolerated and when measured using standardized office blood pressure measurements. Of note, this is lower than the previous targets of <140/90 mm Hg (or $\leq 130/80$ if albuminuria was present) set forth in the 2012 KDIGO blood pressure guidelines. Emphasis is placed on appropriate and accurate measurement of blood pressure readings. KDIGO focuses on utilization of standardized office blood pressure measurements in comparison to routine (or "causal") office blood pressure checks. Standardized office blood pressure measurements are aimed at standardized protocols that include the use of appropriate cuff sizing, proper patient preparation/positioning, proper measurement techniques, accurate documentation and averaging of blood pressure readings obtained.[16] Twenty-four-hour ambulatory blood pressure monitoring is considered the preferred measurement for blood pressure in patients with CKD but is often not readily available and comes with poor reimbursement.[14] The KDIGO 2021 guidelines do caution that it is "potentially hazardous" to apply systolic blood pressure (SBP) targets <120 to blood pressure readings obtained in a nonstandardized manner.[16] Furthermore, target blood pressures for patients with renal transplants are recommended at <130/<80.[16] Potential causes of secondary hypertension should be evaluated when suspected. Etiologies of secondary hypertension include renovascular hypertension, primary aldosteronism, pheochromocytoma, Cushing syndrome, thyroid disease, and obstructive sleep apnea. Causes of chemical and drug-induced secondary hypertension include concomitant use of caffeine, alcohol, nonsteroidal anti-inflammatory drugs (NSAIDs), oral contraceptives, steroids, calcineurin inhibitors, and both prescribed/illicit drugs such as amphetamines and cocaine.[14]

The management of hypertension is first aimed at nonpharmacological therapies such as dietary modifications and weight reduction. The KDIGO 2021 suggests limiting sodium intake to <2 g/day. While the Dietary Approaches to Stop Hypertension diet, including diets high in fruits and vegetables, low in saturated fats, and using salt substitutes, has been found to lower blood pressure by up to ~10 mm Hg, this diet may predispose patients with CKD to hyperkalemia. Moderate intensity exercise is recommended for a cumulative duration of $\geq$150 minutes per week, as tolerated.[16] Weight loss has been shown to reduce blood pressure by ~5 mm Hg for every 5 kg of weight loss.[14] Alcohol use should be limited as well.

Pharmacological management includes the use of renin-angiotensin-system inhibitors (RASi) (including ACEi or ARB) as first-line therapy choice for antihypertensives for hypertensive CKD patients with moderate-to-severe albuminuria/proteinuria, with or without diabetes.[16] RASi therapy reduces intraglomerular pressure and ultimately suppresses proteinuria, offering renal protection to patients with and without diabetes.[14] Combination therapy with both ACEi and ARBs is no longer recommended per KDIGO 2021 guidelines. Second and third-line agents include loop diuretic therapy vs nondihydropyridine calcium-channel blockers (CCB), respective of clinical evidence of hypervolemia. For nonproteinuric hypertensive patients, first-line therapy often includes diuretic therapy if volume overload is present. Subclinical volume overload is present in up to 50% of patients with CKD.[2,17] Thiazide diuretics should be considered first-line therapy for nonproteinuria patients but are often less effective as eGFR falls below 30 mL/min. Loop diuretics are often preferred as eGFR declines.[14] Without clinical evidence of overload, first-line therapy is then directed at either RASi therapy or dihydropyridine CCB for blood pressure control.[17] Resistant hypertension is defined as requiring $\geq$ 4 medications to adequately control blood pressure and is strongly linked to sodium retention in patients with CKD.[18] Diuretic and mineralocorticoid receptor antagonist (such as spironolactone) therapy should be a mainstay of therapy for CKD patients with resistant hypertension.[17,18]

Hyperkalemia

Hyperkalemia is a common electrolyte abnormality of patients with CKD. Untreated, it frequently presents as a serious complication of CKD associated with increased mortality.[19] Hyperkalemia is classified into mild (5.5–6.0 mmol/L), moderate (6.0–6.5 mmol/L), and severe (>6.5 mmol/L).[20] As CKD advances, resulting in a decline in eGFR and subsequent loss of residual renal function, there is a higher prevalence of hyperkalemia as potassium excretion is decreased.[20] Risk factors for hyperkalemia in patients with CKD include associated comorbid conditions such as diabetes, hypertension, heart failure, Type 4 renal tubular acidosis, Addison's disease, and hypoaldosteronism. Use of RAAS inhibitor therapy (ACE inhibitors/angiotensin receptor blockers), NSAIDs, angiotensin receptor neprilysin inhibitors, potassium-sparing diuretics, beta-2-adrenergic receptor blockers, and calcineurin inhibitors in renal transplant patients have been associated with increased incidences of hyperkalemia.[19–21] Diets high in potassium-rich foods contribute to hyperkalemia in patients with CKD as well. Anti-RAAS therapy is often used as a mainstay treatment in patents with CKD for renal protection and preservation, especially in patients with proteinuria; however, these medications frequently contribute to the development of hyperkalemia.[19,21,22] Hyperkalemia associated with anti-RAAS therapy often leads to discontinuation of therapy, which in turn has been shown to negatively impact patients with CKD and has been associated with progression of CKD, initiation of dialysis therapies, negative cardiovascular outcomes and even death.[20]

Patients with hyperkalemia may present with muscle weakness/paresthesia, paralysis, cardiac arrhythmias including bradycardia, ventricular fibrillation/tachycardia and, cardiac arrest. Electorocardiogram changes are often indicated by progressive changes including depressed ST segment, peaked T waves, widened PR intervals, widened QRS segments, loss of P-waves, a sine-wave pattern, ventricular fibrillation, and asystole.[21] Treatment is typically divided into acute versus chronic management. Acute treatment includes temporizing agents (calcium gluconate, insulin, dextrose, b-adrenergic antagonists), use of sodium bicarbonate or diuretic therapy, or initiation of hemodialysis. Chronic management is typically aimed at adjusting/cessation of anti-RAAS therapy, oral diuretics to help potassium secretion, sodium bicarbonate therapy if associated with acidosis, oral potassium-binding agents and potassium-restricted diets.[20] Daily potassium intake of 203 g/day is recommended in patients with CKD who are at risk for developing hyperkalemia.[19] Gastrointestinal (GI) cation exchanging agents are commonly used to lower serum potassium levels. Sodium polystyrene sulfonate (Kayexalate), approved by the U.S. Food and Drug Administration (FDA) over 50 years ago, is often used as an oral resin agent that exchanges potassium for sodium in the gut.[19] It does come with a negative GI side-effect profile, leading to noncompliance, and has also been linked to cases of intestinal necrosis.[19,23] In recent years, newer cation exchange agents have been developed as an optimal alternative for the treatment of hyperkalemia. Sodium zirconium cyclosilicate (Lokelma) and patiromer (Veltassa) have both shown effectiveness in lowering serum potassium levels with generally tolerated side-effect profiles.[19]

Metabolic Acidosis

Metabolic acidosis of CKD is associated with worsening progress of CKD.[1,24] Metabolic acidosis is often common when eGFR falls less than 40 mL/min per 1.73 m^2 and worsens as eGFR decreases.[24] Acidosis is defined as a serum bicarbonate level persistently less than 22 mEq/L.[1] The prevalence of metabolic acidosis in patients with CKD is approximately 15%.[24–26] Persistent acidosis has been found to be associated with progression of CKD, insulin resistance, bone demineralization, skeletal muscle catabolism, and increased mortality.[5,27]

Treatment of metabolic acidosis is aimed at alkali therapy, typically in the form of oral sodium bicarbonate therapy dosing two to three times daily, with a goal of maintaining a serum bicarbonate level between 22 and 28 mmol/L.[27] Implementation of nutritional/dietary changes have been shown to aid in the management of metabolic acidosis. Diets high in "base-producing" fruits and vegetables, with reduced dietary animal protein intake, have been shown to assist in the control of acidosis.[26,28]

Anemia

Anemia is a common complication of CKD, and is associated with poor outcomes including an increased risk for death.[29,30] The prevalence of anemia in patients with CKD increases with worsening eGFR.[31] The 2012 KDIGO guidelines identify anemia based on the hemoglobin values for adults set forth by the World Health Organization definition of anemia. This definition has established a benchmark for anemia evaluation and is defined as a hemoglobin concentration of <13.0 g/dL for adult males and <12.0 g/dL for females.[32] Anemia in CKD is contributed to by multifactorial processes that include relative erythropoietin (EPO) deficiency, uremic-induced inhibitors of erythropoiesis, shortened erythrocyte survival, and disordered iron homeostasis.[29] Relative deficiency in EPO production is one of the primary reasons anemia develops in CKD.[30] Anemia carries an increased risk for mortality and cardiovascular dysfunction, and further impacts quality of life.[30]

In CKD, anemia should be evaluated, independent of the CKD stage, for any potentially reversible causes.[32] Obtaining a complete blood count (CBC) with differential, absolute reticulocyte count, serum ferritin level, serum transferrin saturation (Tsat), serum vitamin B12, and folate levels are recommended as an initial evaluation of the anemia.[32] Frequency of testing recommended for patients with CKD without anemia:[32]

- At least annually in patients with CKD stage 3
- At least bi-annually in CKD stage 4 to stage 5, not yet on dialysis
- At least quarterly in CKD stage 5 on dialysis

For anemic patients with CKD stages 3 through 5 not yet on dialysis, hemoglobin testing should occur at least every three months.[1] Monthly hemoglobin checks are further recommended for patients on dialysis.[32]

Iron therapy and erythropoiesis-stimulating agents (ESA) are treatment options in anemia of CKD, with blood transfusions being considered in patients when clinically indicated by either active bleeding or a rapid drop in hemoglobin levels.[30] Both oral and intravenous (IV) iron are available for treatment; however, oral agents are generally considered only modestly effective in the management of nondialysis CKD and ineffective in hemodialysis patients.[30] IV iron is generally considered efficacious compared with oral forms.[30] Tsat and serum ferritin levels are used to identify iron deficiency and guide treatment regimens.[33] It is suggested that ferritin be maintained above 100 ng/mL and Tsat above 20% in patients with CKD.[34] Iron studies should be monitored periodically with ongoing iron therapy. IV iron is typically avoided in patients with active systemic infections, specifically when bacteremia has been identified.[30,32] ESA therapy is used to further treat anemia in patients with CKD once iron stores have been repleted. ESA is often indicated when any reversible causes of anemia have been ruled out and hemoglobin levels fall persistently less than 10 g/dl. ESA therapy should be avoided in patients with active malignancy.[30] Lastly, while blood transfusions are also a treatment option for patients with significant anemia, their use does not come without associated risks. KDIGO does recommend avoidance of transfusions in patients eligible for organ transplantation, when possible, to minimize risk of allosensitization.[32,35]

Mineral and Bone Disorders

CKD-mineral and bone disorder (MBD) is a systemic disorder of mineral and bone metabolism due to CKD characterized by biochemical abnormalities, increased bone turnover, alterations in mineralization and volume, linear growth or strength abnormalities, and vascular or soft tissue calcification.[36] The presence of abnormal bone morphology on biopsy in patients with kidney disease is termed renal osteodystrophy.[37] The current KDIGO CKD-MBD guidelines were updated in 2017 and recommend monitoring serum levels of calcium, phosphate, parathyroid hormone (PTH) concentration, calcidiol, and tissue non-specific alkaline phosphatase beginning in CKD G3a.[37] In patients with CKD G3a–G5D, the frequency of monitoring serum calcium, phosphate, and PTH depends on the presence and magnitude of abnormalities and the rate of progression of the CKD.[37] The KDIGO (2017) recommended laboratory monitoring frequency for CKD-MBD includes

- Calcium and phosphate every 6 to 12 months and PTH as indicated by baseline and disease progression in patients with CKD stage 3
- Calcium and phosphate every 3 to 6 months and PTH every 6 to 12 months in patients with CKD stage 4
- Calcium and phosphate every 1 to 3 months and PTH every 3 to 6 months in patients with CKD stage 5 including G5D
- Alkaline phosphatase activity every 12 months or more frequently if elevated PTH in patients with stage 4 or 5
- 25OH vitamin D (calcidiol) initially and repeated as indicated by baseline values and intervention

Hyperphosphatemia. Hyperphosphatemia is a pervasive clinical consequence of advancing CKD and is associated with high mortality and poor outcomes in dialysis patients.[37] However, the decision to treat elevated phosphate levels should not be based on a single laboratory value, but rather by monitoring trends of serial results, and there is limited evidence to support the use of phosphate-binding medications in early stages of CKD.[37] Current KDIGO recommendations support lowering elevated serum phosphate levels toward the normal levels, although the benefit of phosphate-lowering medications is reserved for patients with stage 5 CKD.[37] When considering medication selection, the use of calcium-based binders should be limited and aluminum-based binders avoided due to risks of toxicity.[37,38] Dietary phosphate sources should be considered, as additive phosphates are considerably more bioavailable than animal and plant sources of phosphate.[37,39]

Hypocalcemia. Hypocalcemia is a classical feature of untreated CKD, resulting from diminished GI uptake of calcium due to vitamin D deficiency.[37] Hypocalcemia contributes to the development of secondary hyperparathyroidism (SHPT) and renal osteodystrophy.[37] Current KDIGO guidelines emphasize an individualized approach to treating hypocalcemia, with specific attention paid to avoiding hypercalcemia.[37] According to the KDIGO workgroup, the rationale for this is that mild and asymptomatic hypocalcemia (such as in calcimimetic treatment) can be tolerated, whereas hypercalcemia is associated with increased cardiovascular morbidity and mortality and development of calciphylaxis.[37,38] In patients on dialysis, KDIGO guidelines support the use of a dialysate concentration between 2.5 and 3.0 mEq/L to avoid rapid decreases in serum calcium levels.[37]

Secondary hyperparathyroidism. SHPT is a biochemical abnormality that characterizes CKD-MBD and is defined by secondary hyperplasia of the parathyroid gland with a resulting elevation in the levels of the PTH.[40] Higher PTH levels in CKD are associated with increased morbidity and mortality.[37] The pathogenesis of SHPT is driven by several factors, including vitamin D deficiency, hypocalcemia, hyperphosphatemia, and elevated levels of fibroblast growth factor-23.[37] The incidence and severity of SHPT increase as kidney function declines.[37] SHPT can lead to significant abnormalities in bone mineralization and turnover.[37] In addition, compared with the general population, patients with CKD (G3a–G5D) have an increased fracture risk.[37] KDIGO recommendations for the management of abnormal PTH levels state:

- Patients with progressively rising or persistently elevated intact PTH levels should be assessed for modifiable factors such as hypocalcemia, hyperphosphatemia, and vitamin D deficiency[37]
- Calcitriol and vitamin D analogs are not recommended for routine use in adults with CKD staged G3a-5 not on dialysis, except in the case of severe and progressive hyperparathyroidism[37]
- In patients with CKD G5D, iPTH levels should be maintained in the range of approximately 2 to 9 times the upper normal limit. Calcimemetics, calcitriol, vitamin D analogs, or a combination of these agents may be used to help lower iPTH in this patient population.[37]

Care should be exercised in the treatment of secondary hyperparathyroidism: Oversuppression of iPTH levels may result in adynamic bone disease and the use of calcimimetics may cause hypocalcemia.[38] Conversely, failure to address persistently elevated PTH levels may result in hyperplasia of the parathyroid gland requiring parathyroidectomy. Tertiary hyperparathyroidism may also result from disruption of the feedback loop to the parathyroid glands.[41]

SUMMARY

CKD is a condition which impacts millions of individuals worldwide and is associated with complications that pose a direct risk to patient health and well-being.[42] Declining GFR in patients with kidney disease impacts medication selection, diagnostic testing choice and frequency, and management of other comorbid conditions.[42] Patients with CKD are at increased risk of cardiovascular and volume-related complications, particularly in later stages.[2,9,10] Development of anemia is common and symptoms of anemia may confound the management of other acute and chronic health conditions.[43] Acid–base and electrolyte disorders are common in CKD, and require a holistic approach that includes both dietary and medication management.[44] Disorders of mineral–bone metabolism are pervasive in CKD and may range from mild and amenable to dietary modification to severe and necessitating strict dietary phosphate restriction, use of prescription vitamin D analogs, calcimimetics, and phosphorus-binding agents, or potentially even parathyroidectomy.[45] Evaluation for complications of CKD should begin early in the disease course, and continue through the lifespan. Awareness of complications of CKD and adequate management may serve to reduce adverse patient outcomes, improve patient quality of life, and reduce patient mortality. Referral to nephrology should ideally occur early in CKD to allow for comprehensive management of kidney disease and its associated complications.[42]

CLINICS CARE POINTS

- Chronic kidney disease (CKD) is defined as having an estimated glomerular filtration rate (eGFR) of less than 60 mL/min per 1.73 m,[2] urine albumin excretion of at least 30 mg/24 h, or markers of kidney damage that include hematuria or structural abnormalities that is present for at least three months.[4]
- Cardiovascular disease is exceedingly common in CKD; patients with CKD often have atypical presentation and may present with acute myocardial infarction versus stable angina.[10]
- Hypertension is one of the most common risk factors in the development of CKD.[14]

- The 2021 KDIGO guidelines now recommend a target systolic blood pressure goal of <120 mm Hg for all CKD patients with diagnosed hypertension, regardless of diabetes status, measured using standardized office blood pressure measurements.[16]
- Initial pharmacologic management of hypertension in CKD patients with proteinuria should include use of renin-angiotensin-system inhibitors (RASi).[16]
- In patients without proteinuria, initial antihypertensive medication should include diuretic therapy if there is evidence of volume overload or calcium channel blockers if euvolemic.[2,17]
- Thiazide diuretics are first-line therapy for patients without proteinuria, but are often less effective as eGFR falls below 30 mL/min. In patients with lower eGFR, loop diuretics are more efficacious.[14]
- Patients with CKD are at risk for hyperkalemia. However, discontinuation of RASi therapy is often associated with adverse patient outcomes. Thus, use of low potassium diet, diuretics, and/or potassium-binding agents should be considered prior to discontinuation of RASi.[19,20]
- Treatment of metabolic acidosis in CKD is aimed at alkali therapy and dietary modification to include reduced dairy and animal protein intake.[26–28]
- Anemia in CKD is often multifactorial due to disordered iron homeostasis, shortened erythrocyte lifespan, uremic inhibition of erythropoesis, and decreased erythropoietin synthesis.[30]
- Management of anemia in CKD should address underlying causes and may include iron therapy and use of erythrocyte-stimulating agents.[29]
- CKD induces abnormalities in mineral–bone metabolism that are reflected by laboratory changes in calcium, phosphorus, PTH, vitamin D, and alkaline phosphatase levels.[37]
- Hyperphosphatemia should be addressed through reduction of dietary phosphorus intake and the use of phosphorus-binding medication for persistently elevated phosphorus in CKD stages 4 and 5.[37]
- Both hypocalcemia and hypercalcemia should be avoided in patients with CKD. Mild hypocalcemia may be tolerated rather than risking overcorrection of calcium which can lead to extraskeletal calcifications.[37]
- Secondary hyperparathyroidism results from disordered mineral–bone metabolism. Goals for target PTH level vary based on stage of CKD. Failure to manage elevated PTH may result in parathyroid gland hyperplasia and necessitate parathyroidectomy. [37]

ACKNOWLEDGMENTS

The authors thank Danny R. Robinson, Jr., MSN, CRNA, for his editorial assistance and review of the article.

DISCLOSURE

The authors have no commercial or financial conflicts of interest to this article to disclose, nor was funding sourced for this article.

REFERENCES

1. Chen TK, Knicely DH, Grams ME. Chronic kidney disease diagnosis and management: a review. JAMA 2019;322(13):1294–304.
2. Kalantar-Zadeh K, Jafar TH, Nitsch D, et al. Chronic kidney disease. Lancet 2021; 398:786–802.

3. United States Renal Data S. 2021 USRDS annual data report: epidemiology of kidney disease in the United States. Bethesda (MD): National Institutes of Health, National Institute of Diabetes and Digestive and Kidney Diseases; 2021. Available at: https://adr.usrds.org/20212021.

4. Kidney Disease: Improving Global Outcomes (KDIGO) Work Group. KDIGO 2012 clinical practice guideline for the evaluation and management of chronic kidney disease. Kidney Int 2013;3:1–150.

5. Bello AK, Alrukhaimi M, Ashuntantang GE, et al. Complications of chronic kidney disease: current state, knowledge gaps, and strategy for action. Kidney Int Supplements 2017;7(2):122–9.

6. Inker LA, Astor BC, Fox CH, et al. KDOQI US commentary on the 2012 KDIGO clinical practice guideline for the evaluation and management of CKD. Am J Kidney Dis 2014;63(5):713–35.

7. Levey AS, Titan SM, Powe NR, et al. Kidney disease, race, and GFR estimation. Clin J Am Soc Nephrol 2020;15(8):1203–12.

8. Delgado C, Baweja M, Crews DC, et al. A unifying approach for gfr estimation: recommendations of the NKF-ASN task force on reassessing the inclusion of race in diagnosing kidney disease. Am J Kidney Dis 2021;79(2):268–88.

9. Hatamizadeh P. Introduction to nephrocardiology. Cardiol Clin 2021;39(3):295–306.

10. Sarnak MJ, Amann K, Bangalore S, et al. Chronic kidney disease and coronary artery disease: JACC State-of-the-Art Review. J Am Coll Cardiol 2019;74(14):1823–38.

11. Jankowski J, Floege J, Fliser D, et al. Cardiovascular disease in chronic kidney disease: pathophysiological insights and therapeutic options. Circulation 2021;143(11):1157–72.

12. Fau GR, Suhail F, Suhail F, et al. Cardiovascular disease and chronic kidney disease. Disease-a-Month 2015;61:403–13.

13. Tunbridge MJ, Jardine AG. Atherosclerotic vascular disease associated with chronic kidney disease. Cardiol Clin 2021;39(3):403–14.

14. Ku E, Lee BJ, Wei J, et al. Hypertension in CKD: core curriculum 2019. Am J Kidney Dis 2019;74(1):120–31.

15. Goetsch M, Tumarkin E, Blumenthal R, et al. New guidance on blood pressure management in low-risk adults with stage 1 hypertension 2021. Available at: https://http://www.acc.org/latest-in-cardiology/articles/2021/06/21/13/05/new-guidance-on-bp-management-in-low-risk-adults-with-stage-1-htn. Accessed March 13, 2022.

16. Cheung AK, Chang TI, Cushman WC, et al. Executive summary of the KDIGO 2021 clinical practice guideline for the management of blood pressure in chronic kidney disease. Kidney Int 2021;99(3):559–69.

17. Pugh D, Gallacher PJ, Dhaun N. Management of hypertension in chronic kidney disease. Drugs 2019;79(4):365–79.

18. Nagarajan N, Jalal D. Resistant hypertension: diagnosis and management. Adv Chronic Kidney Dis 2019;26(2):99–109.

19. Palmer BF. Potassium binders for hyperkalemia in chronic kidney disease-diet, renin-angiotensin-aldosterone system inhibitor therapy, and hemodialysis. Mayo Clin Proc 2020;95(2):339–54.

20. Watanabe RA-O. Hyperkalemia in chronic kidney disease. 2020(1806-9282 (Electronic)).doi:10.1590/1806-9282.66.S1.31.

21. De Nicola L, Di Lullo L, Paoletti E, et al. Chronic hyperkalemia in non-dialysis CKD: controversial issues in nephrology practice. J Nephrol 2018;31(5):653–64.

22. Gilligan S, Raphael KL. Hyperkalemia and hypokalemia in CKD: prevalence, risk factors, and clinical outcomes. Adv Chronic Kidney Dis 2017;24(5):315–8.

23. Singhania N, Al-Odat R, Singh AK, et al. Intestinal necrosis after co-administration of sodium polystyrene sulfonate and activated charcoal. Clin Case Rep 2020; 8(4):722–4.

24. Chen W, Abramowitz MK. Epidemiology of acid-base derangements in CKD. Adv Chronic Kidney Dis 2017;24(5):280–8.

25. Moranne O, Froissart M, Rossert J, et al. Timing of onset of CKD-related metabolic complications. J Am Soc Nephrol 2009;20(1):164–71.

26. Raphael KL. Metabolic acidosis and subclinical metabolic acidosis in CKD. J Am Soc Nephrol 2018;29(2):376–8.

27. Di Iorio BR, Bellasi A, Raphael KL, et al. Treatment of metabolic acidosis with sodium bicarbonate delays progression of chronic kidney disease: the UBI Study. J Nephrol 2019;32(6):989–1001.

28. Goraya N, Wesson DE. Clinical evidence that treatment of metabolic acidosis slows the progression of chronic kidney disease. Curr Opin Nephrol Hypertens 2019;28(3):267–77.

29. Babitt JL, Lin HY. Mechanisms of anemia in CKD. J Am Soc Nephrol 2012;23(10): 1631–4.

30. Fishbane S, Spinowitz B. Update on anemia in ESRD and earlier stages of CKD: core curriculum 2018. Am J Kidney Dis 2018;71(3):423–35.

31. Hsu CY, McCulloch CE, Curhan GC. Epidemiology of anemia associated with chronic renal insufficiency among adults in the United States: results from the Third National Health and Nutrition Examination Survey. J Am Soc Nephrol 2002;13(2):504–10.

32. Kidney Disease: Improving Global Outcomes (KDIGO) CKD Work Group. KDIGO 2012 Clinical Practice Guideline for anemia in chronic kidney disease. Kidney Int 2012;2(4):279–335.

33. Gafter-Gvili A, Schechter A, Rozen-Zvi B. Iron deficiency anemia in chronic kidney disease. Acta Haematol 2019;142(1):44–50.

34. Affairs DoV. VA/DoD clinical practice guideline for the management of chronic kidney disease in primary care. In: Defense DoVADo, ed. https://http://www.healthquality.va.gov/guidelines/CD/ckd/VADoDCKDCPGFinal5082142020.pdf. Accessed March 26, 2022.

35. Evans EC. Anemia. In: Bodin SM, editor. Contemporary nephrology nursing. 3rd edition. Pitman, NJ: American Nephrology Nurses Association; 2017. p. 387–402.

36. KDIGO clinical practice guideline for the diagnosis, evaluation, prevention, and treatment of Chronic Kidney Disease-Mineral and Bone Disorder (CKD-MBD). Kidney Int 2009;76(113):S3–130.

37. Kidney Disease: Improving Global Outcomes (KDIGO) Work Group. KDIGO 2017 clinical practice guideline update for the diagnosis, evaluation, prevention, and treatment of chronic kidney disease-mineral and bone disorder (CKD-MBD). Kidney Int 2017;7(1):1–59.

38. Cahill M, Haras M. Disorders of calcium and phosphorus metabolism. In: Bodin SM, editor. Contemporary nephrology nursing. 3rd edition. Pitman, NJ: American Nephrology Nurses Association; 2017. p. 403–24.

39. Cupisti A, Kalantar-Zadeh K. Management of natural and added dietary phosphorus burden in kidney disease. Semin Nephrol 2013;33(2):180–90.

40. Eknoyan G, Levin A, Levin N. K/DOQI clinical practice guidelines for bone metabolism and disease in chronic kidney disease. Am J Kidney Dis 2003;42(Suppl 4):S1–201.

41. van der Plas WY, Noltes ME, van Ginhoven TM, et al. Secondary and tertiary hyperparathyroidism: a narrative review. Scand J Surg 2020;109(4):271–8.

42. Inker LA, Levey AS. Staging and management of chronic kidney disease. In: Gilbert SJ, Weiner DE, Bomback AS, et al, editors. National kidney foundation's primer on kidney diseases. 7th edition. Philadelphia, PA: Elsevier; 2018. p. 476–83.

43. Wish JB. Anemia and other hematologic complications of chronic kidney disease. In: Gilbert SJ, Weiner DE, Bomback AS, et al, editors. National kidney foundation's primer on kidney diseases. 7th edition. Philadelphia, PA: Elsevier; 2018. p. 515–25.

44. Bodin SM, Ray T. Alterations in fluid, electrolyte, and acid-base balance. In: Bodin SM, editor. Contemporary nephrology nursing. 3rd edition. Pitman, NJ: American Nephrology Nurses Association; 2017. p. 465–78.

45. Quarles LD, Evenespoel P. Bone and mineral disorders in chronic kidney disease. In: Gilbert SJ, Weiner DE, Bomback AS, et al, editors. National kidney foundation's primer on kidney diseases. 7th edition. Philadelphia, PA: Elsevier; 2018. p. 493–505.

Fluid Overload

Becky M. Ness, PA-C, MPAS, FNKF, DFAPPA[a],*,
Susan E. Brown, MS, ARNP, ACNP-BC, CCRN[b]

KEYWORDS

- Fluid/volume overload • Inpatient • Sepsis • AKI • Fluid restriction
- Sodium restricted diet • Goal-directed therapy • Loop diuretics

KEY POINTS

- Volume overload is an independent risk factor for more rapid decline in kidney function resulting in the need for kidney replacement therapy, including continuous renal replacement therapy, which may be needed in hemodynamically unstable or oliguric patients to address volume overload.
- Goal directed therapy individualized to the patient's hemodynamics should guide fluid resuscitation with careful consideration for the risk of volume overload.
- Inpatient treatment often includes intravenous diuretics, with multiple studies demonstrating that continuous diuretic infusions are no more adventitious than bolus dosing.
- Outpatient treatment and prevention often focuses on 3 main areas:
a. sodium restriction (1.5-2 g for patients with heart failure and up to 2 g for patients with cirrhosis) with recommendation given to follow diet such as the DASH diet
b. fluid restriction is common in the setting of heart failure (1-2 L daily) as well as those with cirrhosis with concomitant hyponatremia
c. daily weights and accurate intake and output monitoring

INTRODUCTION

The utilization of intravenous (IV) fluids is commonplace within the inpatient setting, especially in the intensive care unit (ICU). The fluid needs of each patient evolve throughout their stay and achieving the balance between adequate fluid resuscitation, as in the setting of septic shock, and volume overload is challenging and has been the increasing focus of study within many sources of literature given the negative outcomes associated with volume overload.

In general, volume overload refers to expansion of the extracellular fluid volume. This expansion typically occurs in heart failure, kidney failure, nephrotic syndrome, and cirrhosis. Sodium retention within the kidney leads to increased total body sodium

[a] Mayo Clinic Health System SWMN Region—Mankato, 1025 Marsh Street, Mankato, MN 56001, USA; [b] Southeast Iowa Regional Medical Center—Nephrology, 1223 South Gear Avenue Suite 205, West Burlington, IA 52655, USA
* Corresponding author.
E-mail address: ness.becky@mayo.edu

Crit Care Nurs Clin N Am 34 (2022) 409–420
https://doi.org/10.1016/j.cnc.2022.07.001
0899-5885/22/© 2022 Elsevier Inc. All rights reserved.

content. This increase results in varying degrees of volume overload. The serum sodium concentration in volume-overloaded patients can be high, low, or normal, despite the increased total body sodium content.[1] The volume overload can be associated with altered cognition, altered gas exchange, diastolic dysfunction, cholestasis, intestinal malabsorption, reduced glomerular filtration rate (eGFR), and difficulty in wound healing. Treatment focuses on the removal of excess fluid with diuretics or mechanical fluid removal through methods such as dialysis and paracentesis.[2]

In patients with underlying kidney disease, this balance can be more challenging to achieve and maintain due to the pathologic changes within the kidney. Additional challenges can be seen, not only in identifying the developing volume overload but also the interplay with comorbid conditions such as heart failure or liver disease, which can alter presentation as well as treatment options. This article walks through these presenting disease states, provides guidance and suggestion in the identification of volume overload, as well as treatment options, and how to prevent recurrence. Outpatient management is also covered as this can provide insight on pre- and post-admission challenges for patients as part of recurrence prevention.

ETIOLOGY OF VOLUME OVERLOAD

The etiology of volume overload can be simple, excess fluid in the setting of altered pathophysiology, such as chronic kidney disease (CKD) with congestive heart failure (CHF), or complex as in the setting of multiple system organ failure in the setting of septic shock in the ICU. Regardless of the cause, volume overload has been identified as a risk factor for both cardiovascular morbidity and all-cause mortality, independent of the presence of diabetes mellitus, serum albumin levels, and cardiovascular disease.[3] In patients with CKD, the loss of functioning nephrons results in altered extracellular fluid homeostasis. This loss is characterized by increases in total body sodium and plasma volume. This increase in volume can be seen on physical examination: pedal edema, ascites, dyspnea, as well as laboratory evaluation such as elevated levels of N-terminal (NT)-pro-brain natriuretic peptide (proBNP). There are several factors involved in the progression of CKD in the setting of volume overload as outlined in **Fig. 1**.

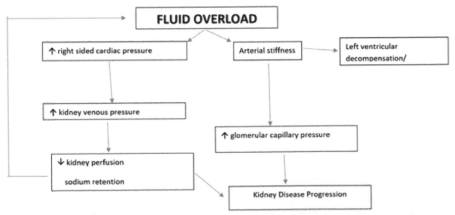

Fig. 1. Mechanisms of kidney disease progression in the setting of volume overload.

Not only does volume overload result in the progression of CKD, but adverse effects can also be seen in most organ systems of the body (**Fig. 2**) including the brain and central nervous system, lungs, cardiovascular system, liver, gastrointestinal (GI) tract, and skin and soft tissues.[4] In the setting of volume overload, the development of interstitial edema precipitates organ dysfunction including impaired oxygenation and metabolite diffusion, obstructed organ perfusion along with venous outflow and lymphatic drainage, and disturbed cell–cell interactions.[4]

CAUSES OF VOLUME OVERLOAD
Sepsis

In the setting of septic shock, hypovolemia results in endothelial dysfunction and vasodilation, which leads to increased vascular permeability and resultant leakage of water into the extravascular space. This process can lead to third spacing of fluid, which in turn results in additional fluid administration that perpetuates the cycle of increased transmural vascular leakage into the tissues resulting in increased organ edema, system dysfunction, and ultimately increased mortality and cardiovascular morbidity.[5] Fluid resuscitation is the primary treatment in patients with sepsis, along with antibiotics and vasoactive agents. Recently vasoplegia has been identified as the primary mechanism in the development of septic shock. With this, the focus on therapy continues with early fluid resuscitation but with caution to identify the optimal amount on a per patient basis, using a rational and stewardship-type approach, like that seen with antibiotic administration. To achieve this optimal balance, close monitoring and documentation of intake and output is critical and nursing plays an essential role in this process.

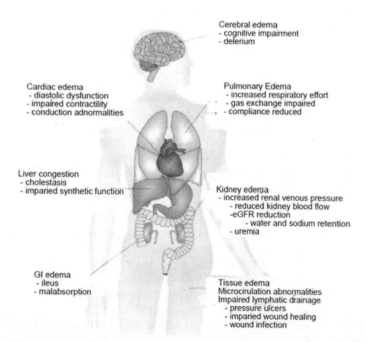

Fig. 2. Systemic adverse effects of fluid overload. (Prowle, J., Echeverri, J., Ligabo, E. et al. Fluid balance and acute kidney injury. Nat Rev Nephrol 6, 107–115 (2010). https://doi.org/10.1038/nrneph.2009.213.)

Acute Kidney Injury

Acute kidney injury (AKI) is not only a cause of volume overload but can also be caused by aggressive fluid resuscitation for other conditions, such as sepsis or hypotension. Volume overload, unlike volume depletion, is a common complication of AKI, especially in patients with oliguria or anuria. Although the association between volume overload and AKI is well known, the cause–effect relationship is less clear.[6] Both volume overload and AKI can result in multi-organ failure and the mechanisms are similar. Volume overload results in endothelial dysfunction due to ischemia-reperfusion injury and inflammation that causes damage to glycocalyx resulting in capillary leakage. This leakage results in interstitial edema, which can lead to reduced diffusion of oxygen and metabolites from the capillaries to the tissues. Interstitial edema also increases tissue pressure, which can result in decreased lymphatic drainage due to obstruction. These mechanisms are what results in multi-organ failure. The kidney's ability to accommodate this increased interstitial pressure is limited by the renal capsule, which results in these changes being more prominently noted in the kidney.[7]

Congestive Heart Failure

In chronic CHF, water and sodium retention in the kidney results in intravascular and interstitial fluid volume expansion and redistribution. Initially the kidney responds to this myocardial dysfunction, prompting additional retention of water and sodium. Unfortunately, over time this compensatory mechanism becomes detrimental resulting in volume overload and congestion.[8] In acute/decompensated heart failure, the resulting volume overload is usually significantly worse than baseline resulting in the presenting symptoms of dyspnea, pedal edema, ascites, and others. The pathophysiology in acute decompensated heart failure is more complex, involving neurohormonal and other cellular modulators as well as interaction between other organs such as the kidneys or liver and the heart.

Using the Brain Natriuretic Peptide and Pro NT-Brain Natriuretic Peptide to Evaluate Heart Failure

Elevated levels of brain natriuretic peptide (BNP) can be seen in volume overload and other conditions such as myocardial infarction, renal failure, obesity, and pulmonary embolism making measurement of a high BNP non-specific for volume overload. However, a normal BNP can exclude the presence of heart failure.[9]

Liver Disease

In patients with liver disease, such as cirrhosis and portal hypertension, progression of the disease process often results in volume overload. In this setting, the vasodilation of the splanchnic vessels results in hypovolemia that triggers the renin–angiotensin–aldosterone system (RAAS) which results in sodium and water retention. This in turn causes vasoconstriction in the kidneys. In addition, splanchnic vasodilatation results in increased splanchnic lymph production to the point of exceeding the capacity to transport resulting in leakage into the peritoneal cavity. This results in sustained ascites, which causes increased intra-abdominal pressure.[10] These pathologic changes can result in AKI that further contributes to the volume overload.[11]

MANAGEMENT OF VOLUME OVERLOAD IN ACUTE AND CRITICAL CARE SETTINGS
Nursing Assessment

Nursing care of volume overload includes initial assessment of increasing shortness of breath, orthopnea, nocturnal dyspnea, fatigue, loss of appetite, weight gain, urine output, mental status, and jugular vein distention (JVD). Bedside testing includes assessment of hemodynamics by checking blood pressure (BP), heart rate and respiratory rate, pulse oximetry, and objective assessment of anxiety. Physical examination includes heart and breath sounds, abdominal distention, JVD, and peripheral edema. As well as providing and adjusting oxygen therapy as ordered.

The nursing role in a critical care setting includes physical assessment as well as measurement of invasive and noninvasive hemodynamic monitoring. Critical care nurses also assist respiratory therapists in managing invasive and noninvasive mechanical ventilation.

Ongoing nursing care includes documentation of daily weight, fluid restriction and careful intake and output monitoring with utilization of indwelling urinary catheter only when absolutely necessary to minimize risk of urinary tract infections. Additionally in fluid overloaded patients, regardless of cause, nursing care includes compression therapy, utilization of passive leg elevation and Education regarding the importance of complying with sodium restriction been ordered.

Sepsis

Volume overload frequently occurs in patients with sepsis. Goal-directed therapy associated with severe sepsis requires multiple liters of crystalloid, colloid, and/or balanced solutions combined with antibiotics and vasopressor support as needed. Hemodynamic targets include a mean arterial pressure (MAP) of 65 to 70 mmHg, systolic BP of greater than 90 mm Hg, central venous pressure (CVP) equal to or greater than 8 mmHg and an $SCVO_2$ of equal to or greater than 70%.[12] Additional invasive hemodynamic parameters may be helpful. Once hemodynamic goals are achieved and tissue perfusion improved as evidenced by normalizing lactic acid levels and improved electrolytes, acid–base balance and assessment of renal function, the process of creating a negative fluid balance and subsequent euvolemia is necessary to improve the outcomes and prevent complications.[13]

Acute Kidney Injury

AKI, much like severe sepsis, often requires an initial component of fluid resuscitation particularly in the presence of hypovolemia, systemic vasodilation, or renal shunting, as can occur in systemic inflammatory response syndrome, severe sepsis, hepatorenal syndrome, hypercalcemia, compartment syndrome as well as exposure to nephrotoxic agents such as Non steroidal anti inflammatory drug (NSAIDs), angiotensin converting enzyme inhibitors (ACEi)/angiotensin receptor blockers (ARBs), and iodinated contrast.[13] AKI, regardless of cause, predisposes the patient to decreased urine output and subsequent volume overload. Mortality increases as the degree of volume overload worsens.[13] The Program to Improve Care in Acute Renal Disease study found that fluid overload was an independent risk factor for increased mortality regardless of the requirement for renal replacement therapy.[14] The Kidney Disease Improving Global Outcomes does not recommend the use of diuretics unless volume overload is present. However, urine response to diuretics in the patient with AKI may be a prognostic factor indicating intact tubular function.[13]

The management of volume overload from severe sepsis or AKI includes enhancing hemodynamics and renal perfusion as needed with vasopressors followed by initiation of loop diuretics. In the oligoanuric and anuric patients, diuretic delivery will be decreased due to impaired renal blood flow. A loading dose of IV loop diuretic will likely be needed to rapidly achieve the peak serum concentration with urine output response determining drug effectiveness.[15]

Acute Decompensated Heart Failure

Acute decompensated heart failure with or without a preserved ejection fraction (heart failure with preserved ejection fraction (HFpEF) or heart failure with reduced ejection fraction (HFrEF) encompasses a rapid onset of heart failure symptoms including JVD, hepatojugular reflex, adventitious breath sounds, dyspnea, and lower extremity edema. The chest x-ray will often identify cardiomegaly and pulmonary vascular congestion. The cornerstone of therapy is diuretics and vasodilators, if hemodynamically stable. In cardiogenic shock, implementation of positive inotropic drugs, vasopressors, and placement of a pulmonary artery catheter to measure pulmonary capillary wedge pressure, stroke volume, systemic vascular resistance, and cardiac index will help to accurately diagnose and guide therapy. In isolated severe cases, intra-aortic balloon counter propulsion and mechanical ventilation are needed for hemodynamic stabilization before and/or concurrently with diuretics.[12] IV diuretic dosing is 2 to 2.5 times the pre-existing oral diuretic dose twice daily to attain a urine output goal of 3 to 4 mL/kg/h. The Diuretics Strategies in Patients with Acute Decompensated Heart Failure study[16] found no benefit to continuously infused loop diuretics compared with twice-daily IV bolus dosing. Furthermore, the same study found that although short-term worsening of renal function was seen when high-dose diuretic strategies were used, at 60 days, the outcomes for high-dose versus low-dose diuretic strategies were similar.

In chronic heart failure patients using loop diuretics such as furosemide, bumetanide, or torsemide administered intravenously dosed at 2 to 2.5 times, the oral maintenance dose twice daily is the cornerstone of therapy. Twice daily therapy both orally and intravenously prevents rebound sodium reabsorption. If severe edema is present, or maximal loop diuretics have not relieved congestion, concurrent use of thiazide diuretics such as metolazone has been found to be beneficial. Once relatively euvolemic and at least 24 h before discharge, transition to oral diuretic therapy is recommended.[16]

Hepatic Cirrhosis, Ascites, and Hepatorenal Syndrome

Ascites is commonly the first indication of volume overload and decompensation in cirrhotic patients. The development of ascites is correlated to a 50% decline in 5-year survival.[16] Hepatorenal syndrome is a late complication for cirrhosis and accounts for increasing numbers of hospitalizations and greater than 45% mortality. AKI and subsequent development of CKD in the cirrhotic patient is often associated with recurring and chronic intravascular volume depletion from fluid shifts to the abdomen and decreased renal perfusion from vascular dilation resulting in hypotension and a rising creatinine trajectory. Volume expansion with albumin 25% and crystalloids combined with vasoconstriction to improve hemodynamics with octreotide and midodrine are mainstays for therapy. Diuretics have no role in this form of AKI.

The cirrhotic patient with chronic decompensation and ascites should initially undergo diagnostic paracentesis then initiation of aldosterone antagonists such as spironolactone with titration of dosing to obtain and maintain euvolemic status along with a 1.5 to 2.0 g/d sodium restriction and lifestyle modifications such as alcohol cessation and physical activity. The recommended initial dose of spironolactone is 50 to 100 mg/d.[17] Long-standing ascites may respond better to combination therapy with loop diuretics such as furosemide with a starting dose of 40 mg daily and adjusted to response. Interestingly, fluid restriction is not recommended in patients with end-stage liver disease unless they have hyponatremia[17] (**Tables 1** and **2**).

Table 1		
With ascites grades and management[17]		
Ascites Grade	**Assessment**	**Management**
Grade 1—mild ascites	Detected by ultrasound	Aldosterone antagonists and 2 g sodium restriction
Grade 2—moderate ascites	Moderate distention of the abdomen	Aldosterone antagonist with loop diuretics and 2 g sodium restriction
Grade 3—gross ascites	Tense abdominal distention	Large volume paracentesis and human albumin combined with dual diuretic therapy. Fluid restriction only if hyponatremia present

DIURETIC RESISTANCE

The goal of diuretic therapy is to decrease edema, ascites, and pulmonary vascular congestion as well as treat hypertension. When these goals cannot be achieved despite the appropriate use of diuretics, resistance results (**Box 1**).

Management of diuretic resistance includes changing from thiazide diuretics to loop diuretics, conversion from oral loop diuretics to IV therapy, increasing frequency of bolus administration of IV therapy, consideration for continuous infusion of diuretics or combination diuretic therapy.[18]

EXTRACORPOREAL THERAPY

Volume overload unresponsive to medication requires use of extracorporeal therapy. Continuous renal replacement is often seen in hemodynamically unstable critically ill patients to improve pulmonary gas exchange, symptoms of uremia in the presence of AKI, management of electrolytes and acid–base status, and to maintain stable hemodynamics. The specific modality is based on availability, provider and nursing knowledge level, and the individual needs of the patient.[9] Slow volume and solute removal are necessary to maintain hemodynamic stability and minimize the need for vasopressor medications. For the hemodynamically stable patient refractory to diuretics, intermittent hemodialysis may well be sufficient.

PREVENTION OF VOLUME OVERLOAD IN ACUTE AND CRITICAL CARE

Fluid overload is a potentially preventable complication and is associated with increased morbidity and mortality in the critically ill. Strategies to prevent volume overload, particularly in patients with shock, is to use a conservative stepwise approach based on hemodynamic parameters and fluid responsiveness with the goal of treating hypotension, tissue hypoperfusion, and monitoring lactate acid levels. Optimally

Table 2		
Common loop diuretics[16]		
Frequently Used Loop Diuretics	**Maximum IV Daily Dosage (mg)**	**Conversion Factor from Oral to IV**
Furosemide	600	80 mg po: 40 mg IV (2:1)
Bumetanide	10	1 mg po: 1 mg IV (1:1)
Torsemide	200	20 mg po: 20 mg IV (1:1)

Box 1
Consider the following variables when assessing cause and effect of diuretic resistance

Verify that the patient is indeed volume overloaded

Verify the edema is renal related and not drug related (calcium channel blockers) or venous vein obstruction (lymphedema)

Verify that all aspects of the primary disorder (eg, CHF) goal-directed therapy are in place

Assess medication and dietary compliance (taking medication correctly and following sodium restrictions)

Assess for poor absorption of oral diuretics or insufficient concentration of IV diuretics due to reduced eGFR or poor cardiac output.

Sodium retention due to various mechanisms such as activation of the renin–angiotensin–aldosterone system and the sympathetic nervous system reducing diuretic responses

Evaluate for diuretic drug interactions including NSAIDs and COX2 inhibitors

---

following 4 phases to stabilize patients with septic shock using the acronym "ROSE":[19]

- *Resuscitation phase*: The goal is to administer fluids using an individualized approach. Having an understanding of the patient's pre-shock BP should direct the goal MAP. If the patient's pre-shock is normotensive, then a MAP of 65 to 70 mm Hg should be the target. If the patient normally is hypertensive, then a target of 75 to 80 mm Hg would be reasonable. At a minimum, an initial crystalloid fluid bolus of 30 mL/kg given in the first 3 hours is associated with improved survival. Vasopressors therapy should not be delayed in those with persistent hypotension and should be administered once the goal-directed recommendation of 30 mL/kg has been met. Ongoing fluid resuscitation in the "fluid unresponsive" patient may lead to volume overload.
- *Optimization phase*: Optimization of hemodynamics and tissue perfusion is the goal of this phase. A fluid unresponsive patient is defined as having no improvement in cardiac output despite appropriate fluid resuscitation. Studies show that up to 50% of the patients in shock are non-responders. CVP and SCVO$_2$ are not sufficient measures to determine fluid responsiveness. Pulse pressure, stroke volume variation as well as ultrasound measurement of respiratory variations of inferior and supervisor vena cava as well as the internal jugular in mechanically ventilated patients have been shown to be more accurate. In the spontaneously breathing patient, using a passive leg raising technique to measure cardiac output, stroke volume, and aortic blood flow under ultrasound is effective. Unfortunately, the technology is not always available to perform these measures. Ultimately, the assessment of fluid responsiveness and clinical evidence of volume overload should guide when to discontinue fluid challenges.
- *Stabilization phase*: Stable hemodynamics and tissue perfusion should be present in this phase. The patients may require some vasopressor support, but titrating doses down should be the goal. Giving fluids during this phase may well cause volume overload. Maintenance fluids are generally not needed as fluids from medication and nutrition should suffice.
- *Evacuation phase*: Treatment of volume overload in the hemodynamically stable patient who has no evidence of tissue hypoperfusion is the goal. Initiation of diuretics after 12 hours after completion of vasopressor support is a strategy in the

non-oliguric patient. Assessment of the CVP and pulmonary capillary wedge pressure may be helpful. Renal replacement therapy should be considered in the anuric patient. Careful monitoring of tissue hypoperfusion is key with fluid removal.

Fluid management should be goal-directed and individualized to the patient with careful monitoring of hemodynamics, tissue oxygenation, and urine output.[19]

OUTPATIENT MANAGEMENT OF VOLUME OVERLOAD

The goal of management should be to prevent recurring hospitalization. Methods to minimize frequent re-hospitalization are the early recognition of symptoms. Riegel and others developed a theory entitled Middle Range Theory of Self-Care of Chronic Illness. The theory of self-care outlines 3 processes that can be used for outpatient management of volume overload regardless of cause (**Box 2**).[20]

Maintenance

The first process of self-care is maintenance that encompasses understanding the value of medication management and adherence to it. This also includes health promotion practices such as dietary and other lifestyle modifications including the need for physical exercise, smoking cessation, adequate sleep, and weight loss.

Dietary changes after discharge from a hospitalization for volume overload could include a fluid restriction of 1.5 to 2.0 L/d, taking care to identify whether volume depletion occurs. Sodium intake should also be restricted to 1.5 to 2.0 g/d. This includes not only abstaining from adding salt at the table or while cooking but also avoidance of processed foods such as frozen meals, deli meats, crackers, chips, canned soups, pre-made vegetable dips, olives, and pickles. The Dietary Approaches to Stop Hypertension diet and the Mediterranean diet have been extensively studied and found to be nutritious, appetizing, and sustainable diets rich in fresh vegetables, fruits, whole grains, low-fat dairy, and lean meat in moderation. Processed foods are limited to absent in both diets.[21] Severe sodium restrictions, however, are not encouraged due to the risk of nutritional deficiencies associated with a lack of appetizing food options. Hypotension has also been noted with severe sodium restrictions.

Other lifestyle modifications include exercise consistent with patient's ability with consideration of cardiac and pulmonary rehabilitation programs based on eligibility, smoking cessation including all forms of tobacco and marijuana, and weight loss with avoidance of severe protein deficiency and muscle wasting.

The ACC/AHA/HFSA heart failure guidelines recommend goal-directed therapy consisting of loop diuretics, RAAS blockade using ARBs, ACEi, beta-blockers with aldosterone antagonists, isosorbide dinitrate, and hydralazine in select patients as needed. Volume overload can be prevalent in stage C and D heart failure with diuretics as a class I recommendation (**Table 3**).

Box 2
Steps of self-care[20]

The Middle-Range Theory of Self-Care of Chronic Illness is modeled in 3 distinct steps
1. Maintenance
2. Monitoring
3. Management

Table 3 Stages of heart failure[22]		
Stage of Heart Failure (HF)	New York Heart Association Classification	Definition
Stage A	I	At elevated risk for HF without structural heart disease or HF symptoms
Stage B	II	Structural heart disease but without signs or symptoms of HF
Stage C	III	Structural heart disease with prior or current symptoms of HF
Stage D	IV	Refractory HF (symptoms despite goal-directed therapy)

Oral loop diuretics are used at the lowest dose necessary to maintain euvolemia with thiazide diuretics such as metolazone used as needed if diuretic resistance becomes a factor.[16]

Use of medical compression therapy for NYHA Type I and II heart failure has been found safe and effective. Compression stockings and wraps to the lower extremities are the methods that are the most cost effective and best tolerated. Studies using pneumatic compression have been done but are not recommended in stage III–IV heart failure due to the increase in right venous return without improvement in stroke volume and cardiac output, worsening right heart failure in isolated patients.[23]

Monitoring

The second process of self-care is the patient's ability to perceive, realize, and understand the importance of the early symptoms of volume overload. The patient needs education for true understanding of how to recognize and monitor for worsening shortness of breath, the ability to assess for peripheral edema, abdominal distention, and the ability to interpret the results of daily weights. A study done by Chaudhry and others reveals that clinically significant weight gains begin to occur at least 1 week before hospital admission in patients with heart failure. One could posit that the results of this study could be linked to other forms of volume overload including worsening ascites and edema in end-stage liver disease.[22]

Management

The third process in self-care is the management of volume overload. Ideally, the patient in this process is using any additional as-needed (PRN) diuretics, calling providers with a condition report including BP, daily weights, and edema while significantly reducing sodium and fluid intake. Utilization of heart failure clinics with telehealth options may be beneficial in these circumstances. Temporary titration of diuretics may be needed to attain or maintain a euvolemic status. Unfortunately, despite the best efforts of the patient and staff, the patient may require hospitalization for administration of IV diuretics and medication adjustments.

SUMMARY

In the critically ill ICU patient, volume overload is prevalent, is associated with organ dysfunction and adverse outcomes, including an increased combined outcome of cardiovascular morbidity and all-cause mortality. The approach to fluid management should include careful attention to the ongoing need for IV fluids, astute observation of the patient's response to fluids as noted by changes in vital signs, evidence of fluid overload on examination, and change to intake and output measurements. Nurses play a key role in the management of volume overload and prevention of harm to the patient.

CLINICS CARE POINTS

- Start diuresis for volume overload in severe sepsis patients once the vasopressors have been discontinued for at least 12 hours and hemodynamic goal parameters are achieved.
- The presence of hypnotremia is the only indication for fluid restriction in the cirrhotic patient.
- Studies have shown no added benefit to continuously infused loop diuretics over twice daily bolus dosing.
- Patient education is key to prevention of hospital re-admissions for volume overload regardless of cause.
- Volume overload is a risk factor for the combined outcome of cardiovascular morbidity and all-cause mortality.

DISCLOSURE

Neither author has any relevant financial or commercial conflicts of interest.

REFERENCES

1. Available at: https://www.merckmanuals.com/professional/endocrine-and-metabolic-disorders/fluid-metabolism/volume-overload.
2. Gomes J, Liliane Pesavento M, Fernandes Manfredi de Freitas F, et al. Fluid overload and risk of mortality in critically ill patients. MDDIMENS CRIT CARE NURS 2019;38(6):293–9.
3. Palmer B, Clegg D. Fluid overload as a therapeutic target for the preservative management of chronic kidney disease. Curr Opin Nephrol Hyertens 2020; 29:22–8.
4. O'Connor M, Prowle J. Fluid overload. Crit Care Clin 2015;31:803–21.
5. Ravi C, Johnson D. Optimizing fluid resuscitation and prevented fluid overload in patients with septic shock. Semin Respir Crit Care Med 2021;42:698–705.
6. Ostermann M, Oudemans-van Straaten HM, Forni LG, et al. Fluid overload and acute kidney injury: cause or consequence? Crit Care 2015;19:443.
7. Patil VP, Salunke BG. Fluid overload and acute kidney injury. Indian J Crit Care Med 2020;24(Suppl 3):S94–7.
8. Miller W. Fluid volume overload and congestion in heart failure time to reconsider pathophysiology and how volume is assessed. Circ Heart Fail 2016;9:e002922.
9. Granado RC, Mehta RL. Fluid Overload in the ICU: evaluation and management. BMC Nephrol 2016;17(109). https://doi.org/10.1186/s12882-016-0323-6.
10. Kashani A, Landaverde C, Medici V, et al. Fluid retention in cirrhosis: pathophysiology and management. QJM 2008;101(2):71–85.
11. Cardoso er al F. Positive fluid balance was associated with mortality in patients with acute-on-chronic liver failure: a cohort study. J Crit Care 2021;63:238–42.
12. Kollef MH, Isakow W, Burks AC, et al. Chapter 3: Sepsis and Septic Shock, . Washington manual of critical care. 3rd edition. Wolkers Kluwer; 2018. p. 8–11.

13. Moore PK, Hsu RK, Liu KD. Management of acute kidney injury: core curriculum. Am J Kidney Dis 2018;72(1):136–46.
14. Blouchard J, Soroko SB, Chertow GM, et al. Fluid accumulation, survival and recovery of kidney function in critically ill patients with acute kidney injury. Int Soc Nephrol 2009;76:422–7.
15. Novak JE, Ellison DH. Diuretics in states of volume overload. Am J Kidney Dis 2021;XX(XX):1–13.
16. Felker GM, Lee KL, Bull DA, et al. Diuretic strategies in patients with acute decompensated heart failure. N Engl J Med 2011;364(9):797–805.
17. Biggins SW, Angeli P, Garcia-Tsao G, et al. Diagnosis, Evaluation,and management of ascites, spontaneous bacterial peritonitis and hepatorenal syndrome: 2021 practice guidance by the American association for the study of liver disease. Hepatology 2021;74(2):1014–48. https://doi.org/10.1002/hep31884.
18. Reilly RF Jr, Perazella MA. Chapter 4: Diuretics, . Nephrology in 30 days. 2nd edition. Lange; 2014. p. 47–60.
19. Ogbu OC, Murphy DJ, Martin GS. How to avoid fluid overload. Curr Opin Crit Care 2016;21(4):315–21.
20. Riegel B, Jaarsma T, Lee CS, et al. Integrating symptoms into the Middle Range theory of self-care of chronic illness. Adv Nurs Sci 2019;42(3):206–16.
21. Wickham BE, Enkhmaa B, Ridberg R, et al. Dietary management of heart failure: DASH diet and precision nutrition perspectives. Nutrition 2021;13(4424). https://doi.org/10.3390/nu13124424.
22. Chaudhry SI, Wang Y, Concato J, et al. Patterns of weight change preceding hospitalization for heart failure. Circulation 2007;116:1549–54.
23. Urbanek T, Jusko M, Kuczmik WB. Compression Therapy for leg oedema in patients with heart failure. ESC Heart Fail 2020;7:2012–20.

Geriatric Nephrology

Debra J. Hain, PhD, APRN, AGPCNP-BC, FAAN, FAANP, FNKF[a],*,
Mary S. Haras, PhD, MBA, APRN, NP-C, CNN[b]

KEYWORDS

- Geriatric • Acute kidney injury • Older adults • Altered mental status

KEY POINTS

- Older adults have a high risk for acute kidney injury (AKI) that contributes to a significant risk of death, increased morbidity, longer length of hospital stay, progression to chronic kidney disease, and the need for chronic dialysis once discharged.
- A person-family centered approach to shared decision-making and prevention and/or treatment of AKI in older adults is important.
- Acute illness in older adults frequently has an atypical presentation which often is acute confusion.

INTRODUCTION

Acute kidney injury (AKI) is characterized by a sudden decline in kidney function that usually leads to a change in fluid, electrolytes, and acid-base disorders (see AKI article in this journal). Older adults have an increased risk of AKI because they are more likely to have one or more chronic health conditions (ie, diabetes, hypertension, and cardiovascular disease), the physiological changes in the aging kidney, medical interventions, polypharmacy, and a serious infection that results in sepsis.[1]

RISK FACTORS FOR ACUTE KIDNEY INJURY IN OLDER ADULTS
Sepsis-Induced Acute Kidney Injury

Older adults are more likely to develop infections because of an age-related decline in immune system function (immunosenescence) and a blunted response to infection increases the risk of sepsis. Sepsis is the leading cause of AKI and death in older adults receiving critical care. However, impaired immunity is not only related to aging but also disease burden. Risk factors for sepsis are being institutionalized (eg, hospital, post-acute care), instrumentation (ie, indwelling urinary catheter) frailty, poor nutritional status, and cognitive impairment. Comorbid conditions that increase the risk

[a] Florida Atlantic University, Christine E Lynn College of Nursing, Boca Raton, FL, USA; [b] School of Nursing, Georgetown University, 3700 Reservoir Road Northwest St. Mary's Hall, #419, Washington, DC 20057, USA
* Corresponding author. FAU CON, 777 Glades Road, Boca Raton, FL 33431.
E-mail address: dhain@health.fau.edu

Crit Care Nurs Clin N Am 34 (2022) 421–430
https://doi.org/10.1016/j.cnc.2022.07.004
0899-5885/22/© 2022 Elsevier Inc. All rights reserved.

ccnursing.theclinics.com

include diabetes, chronic obstructive pulmonary disease (COPD), liver disease, and chronic kidney disease (CKD). Older adults with coronavirus disease-2019 (COVID-19) and AKI have a higher risk of death than those without AKI.[2] So, it is important to pay attention to kidney function in older adults with COVID-19 requiring critical care. The two major causes of sepsis are complicated urinary tract infections (UTIs) and respiratory infections. Even though gastrointestional infections can lead to sepsis this is less common.[3]

UTIs are common in older adults due to mechanical changes such as reduced bladder capacity, involuntary contractions, decreased urine flow, urinary stasis because of enlarged prostate, or bladder prolapse.[4] UTIs and asymptomatic bacteriuria are common in older adults, particularly long-term residents of skilled nursing facilities (SNF) and those who have limited mobility. Long-term urinary catheters predispose older adults to asymptomatic bacteria. Approximately 60% of urosepsis occurs in adults 65 and older and is related to complicated UTIs. Older adults are 13 times more likely to develop urosepsis and have a substantially higher mortality risk.[5]

Older adults are predisposed to respiratory infections because of decreased cough and other protective reflexes, reduced lung elasticity, reduced mucocillary clearance, reduced immunoglobulin (Ig) levels in the respiratory secretions, increased levels of circulating inflammatory cystokines and malnutrition.[4] There is an increased risk of pneumonia in older adults (4 to 11 times higher than those <65 years) who have severe disease, resistant bacteria as the causative agents of pneumonia in residents of long-term care, and longer critical care stay. Severe sepsis is present in approximately 30% of older adults admitted for community-acquired pneumonia.

A common GI infection in older adults in critical care is *Clostridioides difficile* infections (CDI). Older adults are more susceptible due to decreased gastric and intestinal motility, changes in intestinal microbiome, and slow recovery of microbiome after antibiotic use. More than 80% of deaths due to CDI were critically ill adults >65 years. AKI and CDI are major concerns when prescribing excessive antimicrobial therapy. There is an increased risk of CDI with the use of broad-spectrum antibiotics.[6] Older adults who have taken antibiotics, proton pump inhibitors, or corticosteroids within 90 days preceding CDI are more at risk to develop re-infection. Frailty is also linked to CDI as well as a high mortality rate.[4]

Frailty

Frailty is common among older adults in critical care is associated with a high mortality rate; AKI is an independent predictor of mortality, and with frailty this risk increases.[7] Frailty can be defined as a "state of vulnerability characterized by a diminished resilience to external stressors and has been shown to portend great risk of adverse outcomes in critical illness."[7, p. 2] Frailty can lead to falls, disability, hospitalization, and death.[8] The presence of AKI can lead to a decline in functional status that only contributes to frailty. The findings of a secondary analysis of the Optimal Selection For and Timing to Start Renal Replacement in Critically Ill Older Patients with Acute Kidney Injury multicenter prospective cohort study indicated that preexisting frailty before critical illness and having severe AKI was strongly linked to death. Many of the participants who survived acute illness experienced functional decline and worsening frailty within one year after discharge.[7] A systematic review and meta-analysis examined the impacts of frailty on AKI in older adults. The findings revealed that those with frailty had an increased risk of AKI and as frailty worsened so did the AKI.[8]

Nephrotoxic Agents

Some antibacterials have been associated with an increased risk of AKI include aminoglycosides (gentamicin, amikacin), beta-lactams (monobactams, penicillin, cephalosporins, carbapenems), sulfamethoxazole, trimethoprim, and vancomycin.[9] Nonsteroidal anti-inflammatory drugs (NSAID) are effective in treating pain in older adults. However, despite guideline recommendations to avoid use in this population, many older adults continue to take these non-opiate analgesic for osteoarthritis and other pain syndromes. A population-based retrospective cohort study in older adults (≥66 years) indicated that new NSAID use (within 14 days) compared with those who were not taking NSAIDs had a substantial risk for 30-day risk of AKI and hyperkalemia.[10] Statins have also been linked to AKI. Tonelli and colleagues[11] examined the risk of AKI in new statin users (≥66 years). The researchers found that there was an association between the intensity of statin use (high and medium-intensity statin use) and the risk of hospitalization for AKI. This risk was higher among women and those taking an angiotensin-converting enzyme inhibitor/angiotensin receptor blockers (ACEi/ARB) compared with nonusers as well as those taking diuretics.

Surgery

It is not uncommon for AKI to develop after cardiac surgery, particularly in older adults. Comparison between those ≤60 years and ≥60 years revealed that there are distinct risk factors for AKI[12] such as advanced age and preexisting chronic health conditions. The study findings indicated that individuals ≥60 years with AKI post-cardiac surgery had higher mortality, increased risk for stroke, perioperative myocardial infarction, prolonged hospital stay, and were more likely to need kidney replacement therapy (KRT) compared with those ≤60.

AKI is common post-hip fracture surgery and is associated with prolonged hospital stay and increased mortality.[13] The findings of a retrospective cohort study found that there were modifiable and nonmodifiable risk factors for AKI in older adults (≥65) postop hip fracture.[13] Advanced age and heart disease were independent risk factors and preexisting hypertension, diabetes, and CKD increased the nonmodifiable risk of AKI. Possible modifiable risk factors for AKI were longer surgery time, blood loss during surgery, and red blood cell (RBC) transfusions.[13,14] The reasons for risks of AKI with perioperative anemia and RBC blood transfusion are not completely understood; however, some mechanisms that may be related to this are reduced oxygen delivery, worsening oxidative stress, and impaired hemostasis. Hypoalbuminemia that occurs after surgery has also been linked to increased risk of AKI[14] and to poor health outcomes in older adults with AKI.

Contrast-Associated Acute Kidney Injury

It is well-known that contrast-associated AKI (CA-AKI) is prevalent among adults in critical care but what is important to know is there is a higher risk in older adults. Factors that increase the risk of CA-AKI in older adults are lower baseline serum creatinine (Scr), lower ejection fraction, heart failure, and heart disease upon admission.[15] Pavasini and colleagues[15] conducted secondary data analysis of two prospective studies focused on individuals ≥70 years admitted to acute care for acute coronary syndrome and undergoing invasive treatment. The researchers concluded that even though modern contrast media and hydration protocols are used, CA-AKI is very prevalent among older adults and there is a short-term possibility of death. Approximately two-thirds of the sample with CA-AKI in this study recovered to their baseline kidney function within the first three months and their long-term prognosis was similar to those of other patients with AKI.

Polypharmacy

Most older adults have multiple comorbid conditions (ie, hypertension, diabetes, and dyslipidemia), which may lead to polypharmacy. Polypharmacy is defined as being prescribed five or more medications[16] and is associated with frequent hospitalizations, increased mortality and morbidity, and a higher chance of medication-related health problems.[17] In a descriptive retrospective study of patients with AKI who had a mean age of 74 years polypharmacy was found in 40% of the cases ($n = 40$).[18] Polypharmacy has been linked to adverse drug reactions (ADRs) drug–drug reactions, and drug–disease interactions as well as AKI in older adults.[19]

ASSESSMENT

Performing a comprehensive geriatric assessment (CGA) is important. A CGA is the gold standard of care for hospitalized older adults and is defined as "a multidimensional, multidisciplinary process which identifies medical social, and functional needs, and the development of an integrated/coordinated care plan to meet those needs."[20(p150)] There are varying CGA models but common features include specialty expertise (ie, geriatrician, adult/gerontological nurse practitioner), multidimensional assessment and identifying medical, functional, mental, psychosocial, and environmental problems, coordinated efforts with various disciplines, formulation of a plan of care, shared decision-making that involves goals of care with the patient and family/friends (if appropriate), consideration of rehabilitation, and timely implementation of the plan of care, and continued review and adjustments according to the older adult's health condition, hopes, wishes, and preferences.[21]

The CGA should focus on complex problems, be person-centered, pay attention to the person's capacity to participate in decision-making and if the person does have the ability to make informed decisions the clinician should assure that ethical principles are followed, have a link between social and health care needs, and assessments should be carried out with reliable and valid instruments. Not only is it important to assess physical health, but there should also be an objective measure of cognitive status, functional status, that includes mobility and balance (if able), nutritional status, services required, and in front of family situation.[22] Clinical situations that require close monitoring of an older adult for the development of AKI include volume depletion, trauma, sepsis, hypotension, surgery administration of nephrotoxic agents, and identifying risk factors as described above. Kidney function should be assessed upon admission and throughout the hospital stay. The best measure of kidney function is serial labs that include serum creatinine and BUN. However, Scr, as biomarker for kidney function has limitations so it may not be the best indicator for AKI. Age and reduced muscle mass seen in many older adults limits the use of Scr as a biomarker for AKI. In addition, low protein intake can affect Scr and so using this biomarker may be inefficient for early diagnosis AKI in older adults.[23] Other biomarkers that could be considered for early diagnosis and prognosis include neurtophil gelatinase associated lipocalin (NGAL), interleukin-18 (IL-18), kidney injury molecule-1 (KIM-1), and liver-fatty acid-binding protein (L-FABP).[23]

Monitoring fluid status (ie, intake, urine output, and other sources of fluid loss) provides valuable information for early identification of AKI in older adults. Older adults with a sudden change in cognitive function may be prerenal because of absolute volume reduction (bleeding, volume depletion), relative volume reduction (heart failure, cirrhosis) or hypoperfusion (shock, medications). AKI can be related to an intrinsic renal interstitial (acute interstitial nephritis), tubular (acute tubular necrosis [ATN]), glomerular (glomerulonephritis), or vascular conditions. ATN is common in critically ill older adults. ATN can be because of nephrotoxic agents (drugs, contrast, pigments, protein), inflammation (sepsis, lupus), or ischemia caused by prerenal AKI. Cancer risk increases as a person ages and sometimes AKI can be the first indication of urinary tract-related cancers (ie, prostate and urogynecology).[23]

Nutritional status should be assessed upon admission and throughout the critical care stay. However, assessing with albumin and body composition may not be enough because they are influenced by extracellular fluid volume, inflammation, and catabolic acute illness. Albumin may not measure metabolic responses to interventions aimed at improving nutritional status. Despite this albumin is a marker of nutritional status as well as inflammation, hepatic function, and overall catabolic state.[14] Conditions that influence albumin are nutritional intake, specific diseases, and stress/inflammatory states. Serum albumin levels can be affected by fluid overload, so it is important to consider this when using albumin as a marker of nutritional status.

Paying attention to infections that may lead to sepsis is important. Common infections seen in older adults include UTIs, pneumonia, or other respiratory infections, and less common are gastrointestional infections. It is important to consider atypical presentation of illness in older adults who have an infection. The typical signs and symptoms seen in a younger person may not be present in the older adult and if present is often not until the infection has worsened or the patient is septic. Older adults with dementia may not be able to verbalize any concerns. Dysuria a common sign of UTI may not be present in older adults with a UTI; the first sign may be acute confusion and/or urinary incontinence. In approximately 50% of the UTI cases *Escherichia coli* and other gram-negative bacteria such as *Proteus* spp., *Klebsiella* spp., and *Pseudomonas* spp. are the pathogens.

Fever, the most common sign of infection may not be present in older adults despite having bacteremia. Fever is often absent or not very high in the presence of an infection in approximately 20% to 30% of older adults. They may experience obtundation, agitation, poor oral intake, malaise, falls, or hypothermia. The detection of fever in older adults can be serious and requires immediate attention.[4] A chest-X-ray will help diagnose pneumonia but obtaining a computer tomography may help to exclude an underlying malignancy and provide a more accurate diagnosis of alveolar infiltration. *Streptococcus pneumoniae* is frequently the causative agent and those with COPD *Haemophilus influenzae*, *Moraxella catarrhalis*, and *Legionella pnepneumophila* are common causes of pneumonia. In those admitted to critical care, polymicrobial pneumonia is seen most often.[4]

EVIDENCE-BASED INTERVENTIONS

The best treatment of AKI is prevention and early intervention. AKI care bundles may be a way to support early recognition and/or treatment.[24] The Institute for Healthcare Improvement (IHI) definition of a care bundle is "a structured method of improving processes of care and patient outcomes; a small, straightforward set of evidence-based practices, treatments and/or interventions for a defined patient segment or population and care setting that, when implemented collectively, significantly improves the reliability of care and patient outcomes beyond that expected when implemented individually."[25, p.248] Unlike the sepsis care bundle that has substantially reduced mortality, AKI care bundles have not been used a very much.[24] The various AKI bundles that have been tested have included elements related to fluid assessment, identifying AKI and the causes, and evidence-based interventions.[24] Another possible intervention is having AKI nurse specialists who provide education and create a monitoring program for those at risk or with AKI to assure strategies are implemented early and there is a reduction of redundancy in the system so patients with AKI and the treatments are not missed or unnecessarily repeated.[24]

When prescribing medications, it is important to consider age-related changes in pharmacokinetics (ie, absorption, distribution, metabolism, and excretion) and pharmacodynamics (the physiological effects of the drug). In older adults, the proportion of body fat in relation to muscle may cause an increase in the volume of distribution. A decline in kidney function can decrease drug clearance, even when CKD is not present. The half-life can be prolonged, which will increase plasma drug concentrations. The estimated glomerular filtration rate (eGFR) is not a good way to dose medications when AKI is present, and the patient is not in a steady state. Serial labs with Scr to evaluate the eGFR over time are a better way. There should be a balance between over- and under-prescribing.

The best way for drug prescribing is to consider the desired effects and appropriateness of the medication for an older adult. The American Geriatrics Society has tools that can be used when prescribing medications for older adults (Potentially Inappropriate Medications and Beers Criteria). A rule of thumb when prescribing to older adults is go low and go slow and know the desired response and if the person is achieving established goals of prescribing the medication.

Volume status should be closely monitored as well as paying attention to nephrotoxicity and the risk with drugs such as diuretics, NSAIDs, ACEi, ARB, and vasodilators. Individualizing medication therapy by evaluating intake and output, and adjusting drug dosages as per the patient's GFR calculated by Modifications of Diet in Renal Disease (MDRD) or CKD-EPI is important. Both formulas may overestimate the results in older adults so you may want to consult with a pharmacist to assure correct dose.[23] Starting loop diuretics (IV furosemide or equivalent of 80 mg to 200 mg) for those who are oliguric or have evidence of hypervolemia may be necessary to promote or increase urine output. Accurate urine output is important so some patients may require bladder catheter placement. In older adults starting at the lowest dose possible and monitoring the response of diuretics before determining the need for an increase is standard practice. It is critical to evaluate the results of a CGA that includes fluid resuscitation while paying attention to sodium and water overload. The overall goal of fluid resuscitation is to increase cardiac output and improve oxygenation.

In older adults with AKI stopping medications like NSAIDs, ACEi, and ARBs may be necessary, especially in the presence of hypovolemia. Nephrotoxic agents should be avoided, if possible, particularly in the acute phase of AKI. Take time to evaluate pharmacotherapy and pay attention to medications that may need to be temporarily discontinued or require a dose adjustment (eg, metformin, gabapentin, cefepime, morphine). Antibiotic therapy should be individualized while paying attention to comorbid conditions, the need for continuous renal replacement therapy (CRRT), and changes in pharmacotherapeutics as described earlier. It is beyond the scope of this article to present the treatment of CDI, but it is worth mentioning that appropriate prescribing and deprescribing principles should be followed.

The risks of delirium (altered mental status or acute confusion) in older adults with AKI warrant paying attention to and intervening early. The first step in addressing delirium is identifying the cause and individualizing interventions aimed at eliminating/treating the cause and addressing the symptoms. Some of the causes are uremia, hypovolemia, infection, sepsis, and medications. In critical care, anticholinergic and pain medications are the most common causes. Avoidance of antipsychotic medications as first-line intervention in older adults with delirium is important. Antipsychotics can be considered when other interventions (non-pharmacological and pharmacological interventions) have not worked and if there is a risk to patient safety.[26]

Early intervention is the best way to reduce the acute and long-term negative consequences associated with AKI.[27] Those with sepsis-induced AKI have a poorer prognostic outcome compared with those who are non-septic.[28] Long-term outcomes from sepsis-induced AKI include end-stage kidney disease (ESKD) where the person is dependent on KRT such as hemodialysis, peritoneal dialysis, or transplantation.[27] Long-term outcomes have been identified in various studies as being anywhere from 28 days to three years.[27] The findings of a single-center cohort study found that three years after critical care discharge 22% of adults with sepsis-induced severe AKI developed CKD stages 3 to 5 compared with 44% of those who weren't considered severe. Even though the percentage was 50% less in the non-severe group is still very important to have sufficient follow-up post-critical care.[29] Cho and colleagues[28] conducted a retrospective study exploring the clinical characteristics of sepsis-induced AKI in patients receiving CRRT and the predictors of mortality. The authors concluded that age (average age was 64 years), Acute Physiology and Chronic Health Evaluation (APACHE) II score, red blood cell distribution (RDW) score, platelet count, Scr, and urine output of <0.5 mL/kg/h were predictors for 28-day all-cause mortality.

The decision to perform KRT is similar for younger adults. These include the need to manage life-threatening fluid and electrolyte abnormalities related to AKI, pulmonary edema, hyperkalemia, signs of uremia, and severe metabolic acidosis. However, in older adults the decision for CRRT can be more challenging than in younger adults. Older adults often have different values, goals, and preferences for care than younger adults so making the decision about a life-altering treatment can vary. Therefore, it is critical that a person-centered approach be taken where the person and/or family is informed about the risks and benefits of KRT as they engage in shared decision-making about KRT.[30] When KRT is needed in critical care, CRRT is the treatment of choice for critically ill unstable patients, so when providing education about the therapy to family members they should be encouraged to honor their loved ones' wishes as they engage in shared decision-making.

A question the patient or family members often have is what happens if we start dialysis in the hospital, and s/he needs to receive dialysis once discharged. If a person has AKI and there is no evidence of advanced CKD, there is a likelihood of recovery so once they start outpatient dialysis, they may recover and be able to discontinue dialysis after a period of time usually within 3 months. It is important to note that in 2017 the Centers for Medicare and Medicaid Services (CMS) began reimbursing dialysis centers for dialysis services to patients with AKI. The recovery date when the person no longer requires KRT cannot be more than 6 months after the person stated in-center hemodialysis. Having this billable service allows for recovery time before the person is diagnosed with ESKD.

Lastly, but just as important as other interventions, assessing nutritional status upon admission and throughout the stay and comanaging the patient with a dietitian as needed is important. A low protein diet aimed at controlling uremia may not be the best in older adults because they can have a net negative protein balance, particularly if they are receiving dialysis so this must be considered when determining nutritional interventions. Maintaining adequate nutrition is important to achieve an anabolic state in those older adults with AKI who are catabolic.

SUMMARY

AKI in older adults is common and recurrent AKI can lead to poor health outcomes (ie, mortality, CKD that may progress to end-stage, prolonged hospital stays) making it important for critical care nurses to identify and intervene early.[31] At this time there are no pharmacological interventions that can reverse AKI or speed recovery for common causes of AKI such as ischemia and tubular injury. Currently, most interventions are preventative and supportive. There is a desperate need for new models of care that address challenges and gaps in evidence. Considering the risk of mortality and possible long-term effects of AKI, implementing a comprehensive model that moves beyond critical care as the patient transitions across the spectrum of care may be the best way to reduce the negative consequences of AKI. More research is needed to evaluate models of care. In the meantime, being astutely aware of risks for AKI in older adults and intervening early is consistent with best practice.

CLINICS CARE POINTS

- Older adults have a high risk for acute kidney injury (AKI) that is associated with a significant risk for death
- Prevention and early intervention of AKI is key to improved health outcomes
- Taking a person-centered approach to care supports shared decision-making where the person's wishes and preferences for care are honored.
- The first sign of acute illness in older adults can be an altered mental status, fall, and/or acute onset of urinary incontinence

DISCLOSURE

The authors have nothing to disclose.

REFERENCES

1. Wu Y, Hao W, Chen Y, et al. Clinical features, risk factors, and clinical burden of acute kidney injury in older adults. Ren Fail 2020;32(1):1127–34.
2. Yan O, Zuo P, Cheng L, et al. Acute kidney injury is associated with in-hospital mortality in older adults with COVID-19. J Gero Med Sc 2020;76:456–82.
3. Rowe TA, McKoy JM. Sepsis in older adults. Infect Dis Clin North Am 2017;31: 731–42.
4. Esme M, Topeli A, Yavuz BB, et al. Infections in elderly critically ill patients. Front Med 2019;8(118):1–9.
5. Peach BC, Garvan GJ, Garvan CS, et al. Risk factors for urosepsis in older adults: a systematic review. Geron Geri Med 2016;2:1–7.
6. Lee JD, Heintz BH, Mosher HJ, et al. Risk of acute kidney injury and *Clodtridioides difficile* infection with piperacillin/tazobactam, cefepime, and meropenem with or without vancomycin. Clin Infect Dis 2021;73(7):e1579–86.
7. Beaubien-Souligny W, Yang A, Lebovic G, et al. Frailty status among older critically ill patients with severe acute kidney injury. Crit Care 2020;25:1–10.
8. Jiesisbiek ZL, Tung TH, Xu OY, et al. Association of acute kidney injury with frailty in elderly population: a systematic review and meta-analysis. Ren Fail 2019;41(1): 1021–7.

9. Chinzowu T, Chyou TY, Nistala PS. Antibacterial-associated acute kidney injury among older adults: a post-marketing surveillance study using the FDA adverse events reporting system. Pharmacoepidemiol Drug Saf 2018. https://doi.org/10.1002/pds.5486.

10. Nash DM, Markle-Reid M, Brimble KS, et al. Nonsteroidal anti-inflammatory drug use and risk of acute kidney injury and hyperkalemia in older adults: a population-based study. NDT 2019;34:1145–54.

11. Tonelli M, Lloyd AM, Bello AK, et al. Stating use and the risk of acute kidney injury in older adults. BMC Nephr 2019;20(1). https://doi.org/10.1186/s12882=019-1280-1287.

12. Saydy N, Mazine A, Steven LM, et al. Differences and similarities in risk factors for postoperative acute kidney injury between younger and older adults undergoing cardiac surgery. J Thoraic Cardio Surg 2018;155:256–65.

13. Christensen JB, Aasbrenn M, Castillo LS, et al. Predictors of acute kidney injury after hip fracture in older adults. Geri Ortho Surg 2020;11:1–8.

14. Nie S, Tang L, Zhang W, et al. Are there modifiable risk factors to improve AKI? Biomed Resea Inter 2017;5605634.

15. Pavasini R, Tebaldi M, Bugani G, et al. Contrast Associated kidney injury and mortality in older adults with acute coronary syndrome: a pooled analysis of the FRASER and HULK studies. J Clin Med 2021;10(10):2151.

16. Disdier Moulder MP, Hendricks AB, Ou NN. Towards appropriate polypharmacy in older cardiovascular patients: how many medications do I have to take. Clin Cardo 2019;43:137–44.

17. Kimura H, Tanaka K, Saito H, et al. Association of polypharmacy with kidney disease progression in adults with CKD. CJASN 2021;16(12):1797–804.

18. Malki abidi M, Mouna RA, Chargui S, et al. MO403 Acute kidney injury in elderly epidemiological, clinical, and etiological features. NDT 2021;36(Suppl 1). gfab082-0057.

19. Okpechi IG, Tinwala MM, Muneer S, et al. Prevalence f polypharmacy and associated adverse outcomes in adult patients with chronic kidney disease: protocol for a systematic review and meta-analysis. Syst Rev 2021;10:1–7.

20. Parker SG, McCue P, Phelps K, et al. What is a comprehensive geriatric assessment (CGA)? an umbrella review. Age Ageing 2018;47:149–55.

21. Ellis G, Gardner M, Tsiachristas A. Comprehensive geriatric assessment for older adults admitted to hospital. Cochrane Database Syst Rev 2017;9:CD006211.

22. Sporgiene L, Brent L. Comprehensive geriatric assessment from a nursing perspective. In: Hertz K, Santy-Tomlison J, editors. Fragility fracture nursing: holistic care and management of orthogeriatric patient. New York: Springer Publishing; 2018. p. 41–52.

23. Yokota LG, Sampaio BM, Rocha EP, et al. Acute kidney injury in elderly patients: narrative on incidence, risk factors, and mortality. Int J Nephrol Renovasc Dis 2018;11:217–24.

24. Sykes L, Nipah R, Kalra P, et al. A narrative review of the impact of interventions in acute kidney injury. J Neph 2018.

25. Bagshaw SM. Acute kidney injury care bundle. Nephron 2015;131:247–51.

26. Donovan AL, Braehler MR, Robinowitz DL, et al. An implementation-effectiveness study of a perioperative delirium prevention initiative for older adults. Anesth Analg 2020;131(6):1911–22.

27. Harris PL, Umberger RA. Long-term renal outcomes in adults with sepsisinduced acute kidney injury. Dimens Crit Care Nrsg 2020;39(5):259–68.

28. Cho AY, Yoon HJ, Lee KY. Clinical characteristics of sepsis-induced acute kidney injury in patients undergoing continuous renal replacement therapy. Ren Fail 2018;40(1):403–9.
29. Rubin S, Orieux A, Clouzeau B, et al. The incidence of chronic kidney disease three years after non-severe acute kidney injury in critically ill patients: a single-center cohort study. J Clin Med 2019;8(12):2215.
30. Butler CR, O'Hare AM. Complex decision-making about dialysis in critically ill older adults with AKI. AM S Neph 2019;14:485–7.
31. James MT, Bhatt M, Pannu N, et al. Long-term outcomes of acute kidney injury and strategies for improved care. Nat Rev Nephr 2020;16:193–205.

Acute Kidney Injury in the Inpatient and Outpatient Setting

Samuel Realista

KEY WORDS

- Acute kidney injury • Prerenal • Intrinsic • Postrenal • CRRT
- Electrolyte disturbances • Acid base disturbances

KEY POINTS

- One in 5 adults (22%) and 1 in 3 (33%) worldwide experience AKI during a hospital episode.
- Developing AKI as an inpatient is associated with greater than 4-fold increased risk of death
- There are many causes of acute kidney injury in the ICU unit
- The history and physical exam of the patient is used to differentiate the cause and type of acute kidney injury.

DEFINITION

Acute kidney injury (AKI is the abrupt loss of kidney function defined as the rising serum creatinine of greater than or equal to 0.3 mg/dL within 48 hours (about 2 days), or 150% increase of creatinine within 7 days, or urine output of less than 0.5 mL/kg/hour for 6 hours of nitrogenous waste.[1] If the new criteria as established by the KDIGO committee are met, the cause of AKI should be ascertained and staged as follows:

- Stage 1: serum creatinine 1.5–1.9 times baseline or >0.3 mg/dl (>26.5 mcmol/l) increase (or UO <0.5 ml/kg/h for 6–12h)
- Stage 2: serum creatinine 2.0–2.9 times baseline (or UO <0.5 ml/kg/h for >12h)
- Stage 3: serum creatinine 3.0 times baseline (or increase in serum creatinine to >4.0 mg/dl (353.6 mcmol/l); or initiation of renal replacement therapy; or in patients <18 years, decrease in eGFR to <35 ml/min per 1.73 m2 (or UO <0.3 ml/kg/h for >24h or anuria for >12 hours)

The definition of acute kidney injury has changed over time. Originally, the RIFLE Classification system produced the definition of AKI and included three categories of injury and outcomes that were related to loss and end-stage kidney disease. The

Real Health America LLC, 3700 34th Street, suite 302H, Orlando, FL 32805, USA
E-mail address: srealista@realhealthllc.com

RIFLE trial included risk, injury, failure, loss, and end-stage kidney disease.[2] The risk included serum creatinine greater or equal to 1.5 times increase in one week or seven days and had to occur over a minimum of at least one full day. If the rise in serum creatinine was sustained for more than or equal to 24 hours, then this is considered at risk for development of acute kidney injury. If injury is present, the serum creatinine would have a twofold increase. Failure would be having serum creatinine equal to or greater than three times increase of the current serum creatinine up to 4.0 mg/dL. In renal failure, there can be an initiation of renal replacement therapies (RRT). During loss, there is a complete loss of kidney function for greater than four weeks. End-stage kidney disease (ESKD) is present when there is loss that is stand for more than three months. After three months, the diagnosis for the patient changes from acute kidney injury to end-stage kidney disease or end-stage renal disease.[3] We have moved from RIFLE 2003 to AKIN 2007[4] and are now utilizing the most current, KDIGO, since 2012.

Incidence and Prevalence

One in 5 adults (22%) and 1 in 3 (33%) worldwide experience AKI during a hospital episode. This was based on a large cohort study of 312 total studies with 49,147,878 patients (about twice the population of Texas) mostly in the inpatient setting and included nations that spend more than 5% of their total gross domestic product on healthcare.[5] It is even more prevalent in the ICU with 57% of patients with AKI with data from 1802 patients from 97 ICU units in 33 countries.[6,7] Five percent of hospital admissions and 30% of intensive care unit admissions have acute kidney injury (AKI). Twenty-five percent of patients develop AKI during hospitalization. The remarkable statistic from this data is that 50% of these cases are iatrogenic. Developing AKI as an inpatient is associated with greater than 4-fold increased risk of death.[8–10] Age standardized rates of acute kidney injury hospitalizations increased by 139% from the National Inpatient Sample and the National Health Interview Survey. It is important to note that these are diagnosed with patients with diabetes. The rates increased to 230% among those without diabetes.[11–13] The annual incidence of AKI increased 289% in Canadian hospitalized patients with cancer from 2007 to 2014 with 163,071 patients in the study.[14] Eight to sixteen percent of all hospital admissions are AKI. One in seven hospital admissions is due to AKI. Overall, studies show an increasing incidence of AKI.

From 1992 to 2017, multiple studies confirm that the incidence and prevalence of inpatient AKI are increasing. A study conducted by Xue, Daniels & Star from 1992 to 2001 revealed that AKI increased from 15 to 36 cases per 1000 hospitalizations in the United States (2006). Between data 1988 and 2002, the[15,16] study (2006) demonstrated an increase in the incidence of AKI from 40 to 270 per million per year. It also revealed an increase in the incidence of AKI from 61 to 288 per million per year in the United States (2006).[17] showed an increase in the incidence of AKI (4.8% vs 5.6%) in Australia and New Zealand ICU's (2007). In a study done by[18] between 1988 and 2003, there was an increase in age-sex-morbidity adjusted incidence of AKI requiring dialysis (AKI-D) from 0.33% to 0.35% and an increase in age-sex-morbidity adjusted incidence of AKI from 1.1% to 4.1% for cardiopulmonary bypass in USA (2007). Between 1996 and 2003, Hsu et al looked at incidences with all hospitalizations and found an increase in the incidence of AKI-D from 195 to 295 per million per year and an increase in the incidence of AKI from 3227 to 5224 per million per year (2007).[19] found an increase in the incidence of AKI-D from 1.5% to 2.0% and increase in the incidence of AKI from 5.1% to 6.6% (2007). A Canadian study between 2003 and 2007 by,[20,21] found no change in the incidence of AKI-D (40 per million deliveries) and increase in the incidence of AKI from 160 to 230 per million deliveries (2010). A study conducted in the United States evaluating rates of AKI in obstetric deliveries and Callahan et al found an increase in the incidence of AKI from 229 to 452 per million deliveries (2012). A rare study found a decrease in incidence with[22] looking at AKI incidences in myocardial infarction patients between 2000 and 2008. There was a decrease in the incidence of AKI from 26.6% to 19.7% (2012). A Canadian study looked at all major elective surgeries between 1995 and 2009 and Siddiqui et al found an increase in incidence from 0.2% to 0.6% (2012).[23] looked at a cardiac surgery sample group in the United States between 1999 and 2008 and found increase in the incidence of AKI-D from 0.45% to 1.28% and increase in the incidence of AKI from 4.5% to 12.8% (2013).

The outpatient incidence and prevalence were also reviewed. In a retrospective study, 1.4% occurrence in outpatient with an increased risk of all-cause mortality.[24] In another study, outpatient AKI was observed in 4,611 (3.0%) and 115,744 (2.4%) patients in the development and validation cohorts, respectively.[25] Interestingly, COVID disease data were also reviewed with incidence and prevalence of AKI. Twenty-four studies involving 4963 patients confirmed with COVID-19+ showed 3.7% to 4.5% incidence with overall AKI. The incidence increased with the severity of symptoms: 1.3% was noted with mild COVID symptoms, 2.8% with moderate COVID symptoms, and 36.4% with severe COVID illness.[26] In a second study, 1545 charts were reviewed with patients >18 years old admitted to the BronxCare Hospital in NY with a positive SARS-CoV-2 PCR test. The incidence of AKI in patients with COVID-19 was 39% (608), and the mortality rate was 58.2% (354). 42.6% (259) of patients with AKI were admitted to the ICU. Twenty-six patients received hemodialysis during admission. There was a statistically significant association between AKI and age, race, hypertension (HTN), diabetes mellitus (DM), hepatitis C (HCV), congestive heart failure (CHF), CKD, patient outcome, and days spent in the hospital. Of the 608 patients with AKI, 294 (48.4%), 185 (30.4%) and 129 (21.2%) had AKI stage 1, 2 and 3, respectively.[27]

Causes of Acute Kidney Injury

There are many causes of acute kidney injury in the ICU unit. The major causes are sepsis, cardiac surgery, acute liver failure, intra-abdominal hypertension, hepatorenal syndrome, malignancy, and cardiorenal syndrome.[28] There are three distinct types of AKI (prerenal, intrinsic, and postrenal). The first type is prerenal which is caused by a decrease in kidney perfusion from hypovolemia due to hemorrhage, burns, severe nausea, vomiting, or diarrhea; reduced cardiac output due to heart failure, cardiac tamponade, and massive pulmonary embolism; medications that could reduce blood flow to the kidney; and conditions that cause systemic vasodilation such as sepsis, systemic inflammatory response syndrome (SIRS), and hepatorenal syndrome.

The second type of AKI is intrarenal causes of AKI which is comprised of several subclasses such as vascular, microvascular, glomerular, and tubulointerstitial. The vascular causes include renal artery stenosis and atrial or venous cross-clamping. The microvascular group includes thrombotic microangiopathies such as TTP, HUS, DIC, malignant hypertension, scleroderma renal crisis, cholesterol emboli, and preeclampsia. The glomerular causes include glomerulonephritis, IGA nephropathy, lupus, ANCA-associated vasculitis, nephrotic range proteinuria, HIV-associated nephropathy secondary to focal segmental glomerulosclerosis (FSGS), minimal change disease with acute tubular necrosis or acute interstitial nephritis, membranous nephropathy, or renal vein thrombosis. Multiple myeloma and light chain cast nephropathy also fall in this group. In the next group, tubulointerstitial causes for acute kidney injury include acute interstitial nephritis which occurs due to medication, infection, rhabdomyolysis, hemolysis, crystal nephropathy, uric acid, tumor lysis, sulfonamides, protease inhibitors, methotrexate, ethylene glycol, oxalate nephropathy, and myeloma-associated acute kidney injury cast nephropathy. Acute kidney injury that is precipitated by ischemia such as shock and sepsis, as well as inflammatory sepsis or burns can also fall in this category.

The third cause for AKI is also known as post renal causes. This includes bladder outlet, ureteral obstructions, conditions that affect the renal pelvis such as papillary necrosis which can be caused by nonsteroidal anti-inflammatory drugs (NSAIDs) and kidney stones, benign prosthetic hypertrophy, cancers, and blood clots that are found in the bladder. Ureteral obstructions can include unilateral or bilateral kidney stones, malignancy, or retroperitoneal fibrosis.[3]

History and Physical Exam

The history and physical exam of the patient are used to differentiate the cause and type of acute kidney injury. If the history and physical exam suggest volume depletion, it is prerenal acute kidney injury. In prerenal AKI, fractional excretion of sodium of less than one should be confirmed. With intrinsic AKI, the timeline of events and the rate of change in the serum creatinine should be determined. Laboratory testing can also be useful for providing additional information and when differentiating types of AKI. Urine and serum biomarkers for earlier AKI detection are currently under investigation (NGAL, KIM-1, IL-18, and L-FABP). In the urinalysis, the fractional excretion of sodium is helpful for distinguishing between prerenal and acute tubular necrosis injury. Urine dipstick can also be important if there is protein, white blood cells, red blood cells, and casts. With urine microscopy, which is more detailed, the presence of WBCs, bacteria, WBC casts, dysmorphic RBC, RBC casts, granular and epithelial cell casts with free epithelial cells can be identified. With postrenal acute kidney injury, the presence of any obstructions is confirmed. A renal ultrasound is useful to determine the presence of hydronephrosis which can be present unilaterally or bilaterally.

An important trial called the PICARD trial studied AKI in the intensive care setting and was conducted to improve care for acute renal disease. This was an observational study with a population of 618 patients admitted to the ICU at five academic medical centers. Etiology was characterized by clinical criteria but not biopsy. Many patients had more than one cause. More than 70% of the acute kidney injury cases were from acute tubular necrosis related to sepsis and hypertension. Other causes of acute tubular necrosis included hypokalemia, heart failure, hepatorenal syndrome, contrast-induced nephropathy, and rhabdomyolysis. Acute interstitial nephrosis caused 1% of the cases.[29]

Medications

Medications can cause AKI. Often the medications are prescribed as the treatment for underlying conditions and can indirectly change the course of a patient's kidney function. High-risk medications can include analgesics such as morphine or gabapentin, anti-epileptics, antivirals such as acyclovir, antifungals such as fluconazole, diabetic agents such as sulfonylureas and metformin, allopurinol, baclofen, digoxin, lithium, and low molecular weight heparin. All these medications are associated with the development of acute kidney injury.

Once identified it is imperative to stop or hold these medications. It is particularly important then that the critical care nurse or the provider do a medication reconciliation to address or identify medications that could inadvertently create an opportunity for the kidneys to fail. Moreover, there are medications that are associated with causing acute tubular necrosis which is a condition that can cause permanent damage to the kidney tissue. These medications include aminoglycosides, nonsteroidal anti-inflammatory drugs, ace inhibitors, angiotensin II receptor blockers (ARB), amphotericin, cisplatin, and iodinated contrasts. These medications must be evaluated by a provider, especially during acute illness and used with caution so that we can eliminate and avoid acute tubular necrosis.[3]

Acid–Base Disturbance

The most common acid–base disturbance that occurs during AKI is metabolic acidosis. Metabolic acidosis can vary in treatment based on the source and can be categorized into two groups. The first type is characterized by metabolic acidosis with a normal anion gap and hyperchloremia. This type is common when there are gastrointestinal losses in conjunction with renal disease causing hyperchloremia. The second type is characterized by a high anion gap metabolic acidosis which can occur when endogenous acids and exogenous acids are not in balance. Lactate or ketones can cause increased acid production or endogenous causes of high anion gap. Exogenous acids are acids that are ingested or inhaled such as salicylates, methanol, ethlene glycol, iron, isoniazid, theophylline, cyanide, carbon monoxide, toluene, or hydrogen sulfide. A serum osmolality gap (osmolal gap) must be calculated first to determine the cause and treatment. The delta gap can also be calculated to identify the etiology as well. The anion gap may be falsely low with hypoalbuminemia and lithium intoxication. The anion gap may be elevated without acidemia with concurrent metabolic alkalosis related to certain antibiotics such as penicillin. Severe acidemia can lead to decreased cardiac output, cardiac arrhythmias, decreased response to catecholamines, hyperventilation, decreased respiratory muscle strength and respiratory fatigue, and coma.[30]

There is a conceptual model for acute kidney injury. If the patients are at risk for AKI, determine if AKI has developed. If there is no risk for AKI, then reevaluate the risk as appropriate. If AKI develops, stage 1 of acute kidney injury is present and the etiology needs to be determined and the specific cause of that injury treated. If acute kidney injury did not occur, then continue to monitor urinary output, daily serum creatinine measurements, correct hypokalemia, and avoid nephrotoxic agents. During stage 1 AKI, continue to evaluate medications for dose adjustments. To ensure that the patient's kidneys are protected medications need to be evaluated, monitored, and adjusted as needed. Medications should be closely monitored by all healthcare providers with input from nephrology and pharmacology. Renal dosing protects the kidney and prevents it from advancing to later stages of a kidney injury. When stage 2 of AKI progresses to stage 3 AKI there needs to be a reevaluation and prepare the patient for RRT. The risks and benefits of dialysis must be discussed. This can be a traumatic time for the patient and the patient will need a lot of time and resources to be able to make a decision. The nurse can assist during this precious and vulnerable time.[3]

Fluid Overload Predicament

Fluid management in the ICU is a complex intervention. There are many multiple interacting components involved. Volume assessment, clinical impact, and fluid removal strategies that are effective for feasible implementation in daily care need to be evaluated and monitored. As fluid accumulation begins to occur in ICU patients, resuscitation and optimization is the initial phase. It is then followed by stabilization when further fluid administration can be detrimental. Caution should be used when administering more fluids because this phase is when maximum fluid administration has been achieved. The maximum resistance is the phase when fluid administration is no longer therapeutic. The third phase is evacuation when fluid removal will be tolerated. This is an appropriate time to administer diuretics or renal replacement therapy. When the optimal fluid status is achieved, fluid removal is discontinued. The phases are all dependent on time from the beginning to the last phase.[31] Altered fluid homeostasis causes impairment in kidney function, cardiac dysfunction, pulmonary hypertension, splanchnic compartment is a reservoir, endothelial dysfunction, reduction of oncotic pressure is seen with hypoalbuminemia, impaired lymphatic drainage, and a change in interstitial compliance.

Fluid removal is a clinical dilemma. There is a balance between persistent prolonged fluid accumulation and intradialytic hypotension. There is a fine line between identifying a patient in a congestive state versus determining if fluid removal will be tolerated. There are new adjunct ways to assess a patient for improving fluid management. These novel assessments include electrical bioimpedance, lung ultrasound as well as Venus Doppler ultrasound.

Sepsis Predicament

AKI can occur with sepsis in the ICU setting. The 2015 definition defines sepsis as a life-threatening organ dysfunction caused by a deregulated host response to infection. Septic shock causes underlying circulatory and cellular metabolic abnormalities that are profound enough to increase the risk of death. Even though sepsis-related mortality rates have decreased annually from 2000 to 2012, the incidence of severe sepsis per 100,000 people has increased significantly.[32] Less patients are dying from sepsis with acute kidney injury. However, there are more patients who are being diagnosed having sepsis with acute kidney injury in the hospitalized setting. During an episode of sepsis, it is important to obtain blood cultures and start broad-spectrum antibiotics. This is important because of the predicted mortality in the hospital associated with first-time antibiotic use to prevent shock and delay further complications. It is suggested that utilizing empiric combination therapy using at least two antibiotics for different antimicrobial classes aimed at the pathogen for the initial management of septic shock.[33]

In the presence of sepsis and acute kidney injury, it is important to start fluid resuscitation. Either lactated ringers or normal saline can be used. Studies have demonstrated no statistical significance between using balanced IV fluids versus chloride-restricted IV fluids in acute kidney injury in the ICU.[34] A prospective trial with 760 ICU patients comparing the chloride-rich IV versus the chloride restrictive or balanced IV fluids. There was a decreased incidence of acute kidney injury and renal replacement therapy in the -restricted group. However, the effect of balance solution versus saline solution on 90-day mortality and critically ill patients revealed that there was no significant statistical evidence between the two. The primary outcome and secondary outcomes were both about the same, statistically (Yunos et al, 2012). A double-blind, randomized, controlled trial involving 5037 adults in the intensive care unit with the need for fluid resuscitation demonstrated that balanced multi electrolyte solution (21.8%) and critically ill adults did not result in a lower risk of death or acute injury compared to saline (22%).[35,36] The choice of balanced IV fluids versus normal saline should be individualized. Normal saline should be given with hyperkalemia and severe kidney dysfunction. Normal saline should also be used in patients with cerebral edema or advanced liver disease. When fluid resuscitation is given in sepsis associated with AKI, serum creatinine does improve over time and does resolve within 72 hours (about 3 days) following the injury in ICU. In septic shock, Norepinephrine is the first-line vasopressor agent.

In managing AKI in the presence of sepsis, there is a need to focus on the long-term sequela of sepsis-associated acute kidney injury that includes cardiovascular event, stroke, hypertension, and recurrent acute kidney injury. Recurrent acute kidney injury can lead to stage renal disease. These patients are at substantial risk for dialysis as an outpatient.[37,38] Therefore, nephrology follow-up is needed within a week or two after hospitalization to monitor labs. The risk for all-cause mortality and survivors of severe acute kidney injury with sepsis after hospitalization is high without any follow up. Mortality rates decline when follow-up occurs; therefore, the ICU nurse should recommend that the patient and family members follow up with nephrology post hospitalization.

Renal Replacement Therapy

Renal replacement therapy is used extensively in intensive care units. Fifty percent of patients in intensive care units develop acute kidney injury with approximately 25% of those requiring RRT. The initiation of renal replacement therapy is utilized when there is an emergent or life-threatening change in a patient's fluid, electrolyte, or acid–base balance, and unresponsive to medical management. There needs to be vigilance and careful monitoring with regard to trends over time with laboratory tests. The timing of treatment depends on the situation. For example, when life-threatening indications such as severe hyperkalemia greater than 6, or severe acidemia with a pH less than 7.1, life-threatening volume overload or uremia, are all reasons for conventional RRT.

There are several types of RRT that may be used. Intermittent hemodialysis is the preferred treatment for severe hyperkalemia, poisoning, and tumor lysis syndrome. This modality or treatment is to be avoided in patients with intracranial hypertension, acute brain injury, fulminant liver failure, or severe hemodynamic instability. Continuous renal replacement therapy is the modality and treatment of choice in severe hemodynamic instability, intolerance with rapid shifts in fluid balance, intercranial hypertension, acute brain injury, and fulminant liver failure. Continuous renal replacement therapy (CRRT) consists of different modalities for solute clearance. For convection, there is continuous venovenous hemofiltration (CVVH). For diffusion, there is continuous venovenous hemodialysis (CVVHD). And there is combination of both diffusion and convection in continuous venovenous hemodialfiltration (CVVHDF). All these modalities have demonstrated similar mortality and renal recovery outcomes. The only time to avoid utilizing CRRT is when the systolic blood pressure is less than 90 mm Hg. It is imperative that during CRRT that a minimum systolic arterial blood pressure is achieved. Hypotension or low systolic blood pressure must be avoided during treatment. This can be assisted with vasopressors such as norepinephrine. There are indications for the initiation of CRRT. These indications include volume overload, metabolic acidosis, electrolyte abnormalities, uremia, and persistence progressive acute kidney injury. Electrolyte abnormality cases include hyperkalemia, hyponatremia, or hyperphosphatemia. These are clear indications of when to utilize continuous renal replacement therapy. If CRRT treatments do fail, it is due to poor vascular access flow, or circuit clotting.

When critical care acute care nurse practitioners or providers insert temporary double-lumen dialysis catheters for dialysis, it is important to position the catheter to optimize function and adequate vascular flow. Non-tunneled temporary dialysis catheters with a large bore diameter of 11.5 to 14 French catheters are regularly inserted. Right internal jugular vein insertions require a catheter length of 12 to 15 cm. The catheter tip is at the mid atrium with the atrial lumen facing the mediastinum. But not touching the atrial floor. Femoral veins require a slightly longer catheter length of 15 to 20 cm with insertion through the common iliac vein into the inferior vena cava. Left internal jugular veins require much longer catheter lengths of 19 to 24 cm. The catheter tip located is the same for right intra-jugular catheters. It is especially important to avoid subclavian veins. This is the one site that often gives a lot of problems with dialysis treatment optimization when utilizing CRRT machines.[39] Once treatments commence, it is important to determine the net ultrafiltration (UF) goal for each treatment. If the provider determines that a patient requires more fluid removal, then the net UF goal will need to be a net negative. If the input is equal to the output, then the net UF goal will need to be net even. If the provider determines that the patient needs to be volume resuscitated, then there needs to be a net UF goal of net positive. Intake and output in the intensive care unit can be measured in 24-hour comparisons or hourly comparisons (Nerya et al, 2021).

Anticoagulation for optimal CRRTs circuit function is necessary in some cases. Anticoagulation is often needed in COVID-19 infections. However, CRRT can be performed without the use of anticoagulation. Without the use of anticoagulation there are setbacks decreasing the filter life and inadequate delivered dose of CRRT. Without the use of anticoagulation or insufficient anticoagulation, hemofilter clots, circuit system clots can occur. Unfractionated heparin as well as citrate can be used for anticoagulation during CRRT treatments. The advantage of unfractionated heparin includes its effectiveness, widely available, simple monitoring of partial thromboplastin time (PTT), reverses with protamine, inexpensive, and short half-life. The disadvantages of unfractionated heparin include systemic bleeding, unpredictable kinetics, PTT unreliability for bleeding, low patient antithrombin for heparin resistance, and HIT. For citrate, the advantages include regional use, avoidance of bleeding, adds value as a buffer, and no thrombocytopenia. The disadvantages of citrate utilization are metabolic complications and complex protocols. Complexity can add to the difficulty, challenge to treat, executing the plan, and can cause toxicity. Signs of toxicity include increasing anion gap, worsening metabolic acidosis, falling ionized calcium levels, and escalating calcium infusion requirements to maintain ionized calcium levels within a normal range. Moreover, CRRT is the renal replacement therapy of choice in hemodynamically unstable critically ill patients in the intensive care units and those who are hemodynamically stable and significantly volume overloaded.

In a retrospective study out of 210 ICU patients with acute kidney injury stage 1, Raimundo et. al.,[40] found that an increase in fluid administration after early AKI is associated with less renal recovery. Raimundo also found increased fluid gain in the patients with stage one AKI. increased risk for progression to stage three. Fluid intake then rather than the reduction of urine output was seen as an independent association with progression to AKI stage 3. As demonstrated by the PICARD study, fluid overload was directly associated with poor outcomes in patients with AKI and there was a twofold increase in mortality. Duration and correction of fluid overload influence mortality rates. The more fluid-positive patients have a significant increase in mortality compared to hypovolemic patients.[41,42] Patients with fluid overload greater than 10% weight gain at the initiation of RRT had an increased risk for 90-day mortality.[43] This increased risk for 90-day mortality was noted after adjusting for disease severity, time of RRT initiation, RRT modality, and severe sepsis.

Studies suggest that fluid overload greater than 10% is associated with worsening organ dysfunction and mortality with AKI. Ways to avoid and manage fluid overload include conservative fluid management, diuretic utilization as well as mechanical fluid removal with CRRT. While the timing and best method of removing fluid for fluid overload during CERT are still unknown. More studies need to be conducted and more randomized control trials are needed to determine how fluid management strategies including timing and volume removal in critically ill patients with AKI will affect outcomes.

SUMMARY

AKI is an all-encompassing topic in renal care as well as critical care. Critical care nurses have so much impact on the identification and management of AKI. AKI has undergone changes in its definition evolving from the RIFLE, to AKIN, and now, KDIGO. The incidence and prevalence of inpatient AKI are increasing. It is significant as well in the outpatient setting. There are many causes of AKI and identifying the cause is key in reversing and controlling the progression of disease. Metabolic acidosis, fluid overload, and sepsis require detailed evaluation to best provide the most appropriate plan and execution. Lastly, renal replacement therapy is a remarkable tool that requires expertise from the critical nurse. Once it is mastered, the most vulnerable patient in the ICU can become the recipient of good and positive outcomes. ICU nurses are truly magicians in every hospital. Thank you for all that you do and are yet to do for our patients.

DISCLOSURE

The author has no disclosures

CLINICS CARE POINTS

- Monitor urine output and document carefully
- Avoid nephrotoxins

REFERENCES

1. International Society of Nephrology. Summary of recommendation statements. Kidney Int Suppl 2011;2(1):8–12.
2. Bellomo R, et al. Acute renal failure – definition, outcome measures, animal models, fluid therapy and information technology needs: the Second International Consensus Conference of the Acute Dialysis Quality Initiative (ADQI) Group. Critical Care 2004;8:R204–12.
3. Moore PK, Hsu RK, Liu KD. Management of Acute Kidney Injury: Core Curriculum 2018 American. J Kidney Dis 2018;72(1):136–48.
4. Mehta RL, et al. Acute Kidney Injury Network: report of an initiative to improve outcomes in acute kidney injury. Critical Care 2007;11:R31.
5. Susantitaphong P, et al. World Incidence of AKI; A Meta-Analysis. Clinical Journal of the American Society of Nephrology 2013;8(9):1482.
6. Hoste EA, et al. Epidemiology of acute kidney injury in critically ill patients; the multinational AKI-EPI study. Intensive Care Med 2015;41(8):1411–23.
7. Hsu C, McCulloch C, Fan D, et al. Community-based incidence of acute renal failure. Kidney Int 2007;72(2):208–12.
8. Wang HE, Muntner P, Chertow GM, et al. Acute kidney injury and mortality in hospitalized patients. Am J Nephrol 2012;35(4):349–55.
9. Sawhney S, et al. Intermediate and Long-term Outcomes of Survivors of Acute Kidney Injury Episodes: A Large Population-Based Cohort Study. Am J Kidney Dis 2017;69(1):18–28.
10. Siddiqui NF, Coca SG, Devereaux PJ. Secular trends in acute dialysis after elective major surgery—1995 to 2009. Can Med Assoc J 2012;184(11):1237–45.

11. Pavkov ME, Harding JL, Burrows NR. Trends in Hospitalizations for Acute Kidney Injury – United States, 2000-2014 Kidney Injury – United States, 2000-2014. MMMR Morbidity Weekly 2018;67(10):289.
12. Pratha M, Chao J. Acute Kidney Injury. Five Minute Consult. Obtained March 2020;16:2022.
13. Prowle JR, et al. Fluid Balance and Acute Kidney Injury. Nature Reviews Nephrology 2010;6:107–15.
14. Kitchlu A, et al. Acute Kidney Injury in Patients Receiving Systemic Treatment for Cancer: A Population-Based Cohort Study. Journal of the National Cancer Institute 2019;111(7):727–36.
15. Waikar SS, Curhan GC, Wald R, McCarthy EP, Chertow GM. Declining mortality in patients with acute renal failure, 1988 to 2002. J Am Soc Nephrol 2006;17(4): 1143–50.
16. Xue JL, Daniels F, Star RA. Incidence and mortality of acute renal failure in Medicare beneficiaries, 1992 to 2001 beneficiaries, 1992 to 2001. J Am Soc Nephrol 2006;17:1135–42.
17. Bagshaw SM, George C, Bellomo R. Changes in the incidence and outcome for early acute kidney injury in a cohort of Australian intensive care units. Critical Care 2007;11:R68.
18. Swaminathan M, Shaw AD, Phillips-Bute BG. Trends in acute renal failure associated with coronary artery bypass graft surgery in the United States. Crit Care Med 2007;35(10):2286–91.
19. Thakar CV, Worley S, Arrigain S, Yared J, Paganini EP. Improved survival in acute kidney injury after cardiac surgery. American Journal Kidney Disease 2007;50(5): 703–11.
20. Liu S, et al. Temporal trends and regional variations in severe Maternal morbidity in Canada, 2003 to 2007. J Obstet Gynaecol Can 2010;32(9):847–55.
21. Luciano R, Moeckel G. Update on the Native Kidney Biopsy: Core Curriculum 2019. American Journal Kidney Disease 2019;73:404–15.
22. Amin AP, Salisbury AC, McCullough PA. Trends in the incidence of acute kidney injury in patients hospitalized with acute myocardial infarction. Arch Intern Med 2012;172(3):246–53.
23. Lenihan CR, Montez-Rath ME, Mora Mangano CT, Chertow GM, Winkelmayer WC. Trends in acute kidney injury, associated use of dialysis, and mortality after cardiac surgery, 1999 to 2008. Annals of Thoracic Surgery 2013; 95(1):20–8.
24. Leither MD, et al. The impact of outpatient acute kidney injury on mortality and chronic kidney disease: a retrospective cohort study. Nephrology Dialysis Transplantation 2019;34(3):493–501.
25. Murphy D, Reule S, Vock D, Drawz P. Acute Kidney Injury in the Outpatient Setting: Developing and Validating a Risk Prediction Model. Kidney Medicine Journal 2021;4(1).
26. Yang X, et al. Prevalence and impact of acute renal impairment on COVID-19: a systematic review and meta-analysis. Critical Care 2020;24(1):356.
27. Bandelac L, Shah KD, Purmessur P, Ghazanfar H, Nasr R. Acute Kidney Injury Incidence, Stage, and Recovery in Patients with COVID-19. International Journal of Nephrology and Renovascular Disease 2022;15:77–83.
28. Griffin B, et al. Critical Care Nephrology: Core Curriculum 2020. American Journal Kidney Disease 2020;75:435–52.
29. Mehta RL, et al. Spectrum of acute renal failure in the intensive care experience. Kidney Int 2004;66(4):1673.

30. Androgue HJ, Madias NE. Management of life-threatening acid-base disorders. Parts. New England Journal of Medicine 1998;338(1):26–34.
31. Hoste EA, et al. Four phases of intravenous fluid therapy: a conceptual model. Br J Anaesth 2014;113(5):740–7.
32. Stoller J, et al. Epidemiology of Severe Sepsis: 2008-2012. J Crit Care 2016;31: 58–62.
33. Rhodes A, et al. Surviving Sepsis Campaign: International Guidelines for Management of Sepsis and Septic Shock: 2016. Critical Care Medicine 2017;45: 486–552.
34. Yunos N, et al. Association Between a Chloride-Liberal vs Chloride-Restrictive Intravenous Fluid Administration Strategy and Kidney Injury in Critically Ill Adults. JAMA 2012;308: 1566–72.
35. Finfer S, et al. Balanced Multielectrolyte Solution versus Saline in Critically Ill Adults. N Eng J Medicine 2022;386:815–26.
36. Gladziwa U, et al. Chronic hypokaelemia of adults: Gitelman's syndrome is frequent but classical Bartter's syndrome is rare. Nephrology Dialysis Transplantation 1995;10(9):1607.
37. Silver S, et al. Follow-up Care in Acute Kidney Injury: Lost in Translation. Advances Chronic Kidney Disease 2017;24:246–52.
38. Singer M, et al. The Third International Consensus Definitions for Sepsis and Septic Shock (Sepsis-3). JAMA 2016;315:801–10.
39. Neyra JA, et al. How To Prescribe And Troubleshoot Continuous Renal Replacement Therapy: A Case-Based Review. Kidney 360 2021;2:371–84.
40. Raimundo M, et al. Increased Fluid Administration After Early Acute Kidney Injury is Associated with Less Renal Recovery. SHOCK 2015;44(5):431–7.
41. Bouchard J, et al. Fluid accumulation, survival and recovery of kidney function in critically ill patients with acute kidney injury. Kidney Int 2009;76(4):422–7.
42. Callaghan WM, Creanga AA, Kuklina EV. Severe maternal morbidity among delivery and postpartum hospitalizations in the United States. Obstetrics Gynecology 2012;120(5):1029–36.
43. Vaara ST, et al. Fluid overload is associated with an increased risk for 90-day mortality in critically ill patients with renal replacement therapy: data from the prospective FINNAKI study. Critical Care Medicine 2012;16(5):1–11.

Optimizing Care in Kidney Transplantation

Kimberly Horka, AGPCNP-BC

KEYWORDS

- Transplant • Kidney • Chronic kidney disease • Post-transplant
- Transplant complications • End-stage renal disease

KEY POINTS

- Chronic Kidney Disease and End-Stage Renal Failure is a major health concern in the United States.
- The disease process and complexity of patients dealing with renal disease impacts overall health and length of life as well as health care costs for Medicare.
- Kidney transplantation is the goal standard of care for end-stage patients; however, it is not always attainable.
- Complex health care management of transplant patients takes many disciplines and knowledgeable clinical staff.
- Medical management and special care will be life long after the transplant.

INTRODUCTION

There is a worldwide epidemic that no one seems to talk about outside of health care. Jack and Philip state[1] "CKD emerges to be a global health challenge, there is no simple solution to the CKD epidemic" (p. 119). Kidney failure is extremely prevalent in the US, with many people suffering from chronic kidney disease (CKD) without realizing it. A person can lose up to 75% of their function before having symptoms. It is found that renal disease, or CKD, affects approximately one in seven, or about 15% of all adults in the United States.[2–4] The prevalence of the renal disease is growing as time goes on due to the growing prevalence of hypertension and diabetes in general population, as these are the primary causes of end-stage renal disease (ESRD). There are multiple treatment options for CKD, such as hemodialysis and peritoneal dialysis, but the best outcomes and longevity of life come from transplantation. If a person reaches ESRD and does not choose one of these options, it leads to death.

5333 McAuley Dr, Suite 4003, Ypsilanti, MI 48197, USA
E-mail address: kmhorka@gmail.com

Crit Care Nurs Clin N Am 34 (2022) 443–451
https://doi.org/10.1016/j.cnc.2022.08.003
0899-5885/22/© 2022 Elsevier Inc. All rights reserved.

ccnursing.theclinics.com

TRANSPLANT STATISTICS

Transplant is the best treatment option for a patient suffering from ESRD **Fig. 1**. A transplanted kidney will be the closest thing to a native kidney for a patient. The kidneys have multiple jobs in the body that are hard to duplicate with dialysis and medication management. A kidney not only creates and concentrates urine, but also removes waste and extrafluid from the body, helps with blood pressure management and red blood cell production, balances the pH of blood, affects bone health, and maintains electrolyte and mineral balances. Transplant, however, is unfortunately the less accessible option due to organ shortages and other barriers such as comorbid health conditions in the patient population who would require this surgery. These things can lead to delay or disqualification of this option for patients. The first successful kidney transplant was done in 1954. Since then, scientists and surgeons have come a long way with organ transplantation. The United Network for Organ Sharing (UNOS) helps coordinate organ donation across the country and is the only organization in the United States for this purpose. Congress established this program in 1984 in hopes that organ allocation would be fair, equitable, and efficient. Before this program was established, an organ donor's precious gifts were not able to be used if a match was not found locally in a timely manner. This organization helps facilitate all organ transplant programs in the United States to communicate and ensure limited waste of useful organs.

Deceased donors are more common than live donor transplants and are about three times more likely to be used. The list for organ donation after death in each state varies, and many people on the list end up not being eligible to donate after death depending on the cause of death. According to a 2018 data collection on organ donors per state[4]- Texas had the lowest number of registered donors at 32% and Colorado had the most at 69%. Though these numbers look good, UNOS reports only about 20,000 or so donors for 2021. The US Department of Health states that one donor can save up to eight lives with organ donation after death (US Department of Health and Human Services, 2022). Thankfully, the number of transplants being performed is directly proportional in growth as the incidence of renal disease rises.[2] The organ shortage leaves many patients waiting in excess of 5 years waiting for their chance to receive this life-saving opportunity. Unfortunately, the longer the patient waits,

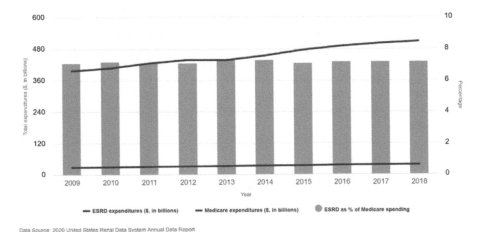

Data Source: 2020 United States Renal Data System Annual Data Report

Fig. 1. Unadjusted total Medicare and ESRD fee-for-service spending, and ESRD spending as a percentage of Medicare fee-for-service spending, 2009–2018.

the more likely they are to have undesirable medical changes that can lead to them is no longer a candidate for transplantation such as heart attack or stroke. Patients on dialysis have about a 5-year life expectancy and have the highest risk of cardiovascular events being their sudden death cause. Any worsening of congestive heart failure, ejection fraction, or new-onset atrial fibrillation can also result in the patient being removed from the transplant list.

Live donors can help increase the number of kidney transplants performed, as well as outcomes for patients, although they are many barriers that make this more limited than deceased donors. People are often reluctant to donate even after death, so finding willing live donors can be difficult. There are multiple reasons people decline being an organ donor, including- but not limited to: religion, faith-based beliefs, lack of knowledge on the process, misinformation about care if in intensive care unit or near-death situations and being a donor, and even just naivety of the need. Even with these barriers, UNOS reports a 34% increase in the deceased donation of organs over the last 5 years (UNOS, 2021). According to,[5,6] there are about 786,000 people with ESRD with 76% of these people on dialysis and 29% living with a kidney transplant. In January 2021, the US government has started initiatives that drive for higher numbers of transplant and home dialysis patients rather than the typical in center hemodialysis setting. The United States performed 22,817 kidney transplants in 2020.[5] The sad reality of ESRD is that many who are on dialysis are not even eligible for a transplant and will never be. Medical diagnoses' such as certain cancer types, such as myeloma, or restrictive lung disease, amyloid disorders, central neurodegenerative diseases, or cirrhosis are not even recommended to be referred for transplant consideration.[7] Those who are fortunate enough to get listed for transplant and then receive an organ depend on the care given to them. Care must be superb to help improve the outcome of the surgery. Being prudent in the care given postoperatively will help ensure the success of the ever-so-precious organ donation surgery that just took place.

The United States has an organ shortage that is clearly documented by statistics. There are approximately 106,600 people waiting for organ transplants in the United States. Of those, about 90,000 are kidney transplant needs.[8] The average wait for a kidney is currently 3 to 5 years, according to the American Kidney foundation (2022). Although there are some research advances in progress with the artificial kidney and genetically modified pig organ transplants, scientists are still years away from these realistically touching the patients in need. These treatment options need to undergo many more years of testing and then get approved for human research as well as how insurance coverage will work. Medicare currently spends a large portion of their budget on ESRD and kidney disease, as they cover ESRD patient care and hemodialysis. There is a large push and some recent incentives to ensure better treatment plans and options to reduce cost, which has continued to rise over the past few years.[9] Ensuring care of the organ post-surgery is a vital step in recovery and will help with Medicare costs as keeping someone off dialysis is not only better for the patient but reduces the cost burden to Medicare. Medicare estimated that they spent 10.3 billion in 2020 on end-stage renal patients alone.

CARE OF THE ORGAN TRANSPLANT PATIENT

Now that we have determined transplant is our best option, we must now discuss proper management to ensure the organ now is taken care of and lasts as long as it can. Studies show that an average deceased donor kidney lasts approximately 10 to 15 years, and a live donor lasts approximately 15 to 20 years.[10] As stated by,[11]

"The care of kidney transplant recipients can be divided into two phases" (p 1). The first phase is early postoperative care. It is the time frame directly after transplant until approximately 3 to 6 months postoperatively.

During this time ensuring optimization of graft function, reducing the risk of and acknowledging acute rejection, and preventing opportunistic infection are most important.[11] Research shows the clinical significance of how this time frame affects a patient long term, as insults that occur within this time frame or up to the first year can impact the length of graft survival.[12]

The second phase is the maintenance of care 3 months postoperatively until graft function declines or the lifespan of the donated organ is over, or death of the patient occurs. During this period, the focus of care shifts to preserving graft function, continuing to get the patient to adhere to a medication regimen and healthy lifestyle, and reducing unfortunate side effects of long-term immunosuppression such as infection, cancer, or cardiovascular disease. For transplant recipients, health care needs will be lifelong.

In preparation for surgery, the patient must undergo a plethora of testing as a workup to determine they are safe for the operation. This surgery tends to take anywhere from two to 4 h when the patient is under anesthesia therefore the patient heart and lungs must be healthy to endure this. Surgery pretesting consists of lab work that looks at the liver function, pulmonary function testing, electrocardiogram, immunogenetics testing (human leukocyte antigen testing), as well as cancer screenings such as but not limited to-chest X-ray, mammogram, pap smear, pelvic examinations, prostate checks, and PSA levels.[13] Often a computed tomography of the abdomen or ultrasound may be ordered to evaluate vascular health as well. Most patients must also follow-up with stress testing, echo, and cardiology clearance. Patients are also recommended to be up to date on vaccinations. Some programs require now that patients are coronavirus disease-2019 vaccinated as the ongoing pandemic has been a large threat to the immunocompromised population.

After initial testing is done, the patient must prepare for surgery with several other things. The approval for a person to be listed on the transplant list does not only apply to physical health. They also screen for depression, social support systems, financial aspects, and insurance as well as past compliance with medical treatments such as dialysis. Once a patient is qualified to list, and they complete the testing required, they are listed. The patient must get on the list before they can have a live donor come for testing to be considered a donor. If a live donor is available then they must also qualify as a donor by a full medical, social, and mental health workup. The entire process can take months.

The Kidney Disease Outcomes Quality Initiative, or KDOQI, is the National Kidney Foundation clinical guidelines for patients with renal disease. This program helps provide a large amount of quality care performance suggestions. KDOQI gives guidelines for management on how a kidney transplant can achieve its best outcome. Preoperatively the guidelines suggest that the patient start immunosuppression before surgery.[11] This is also referred to as induction therapy for medication. Interleukin 2 receptor antagonists are first line for immunosuppression but are advised to be used in combination with another immunosuppressant therapy.[14] An interleukin 2 receptor antagonist drug can be given orally if is a planned surgery, or intravenous (IV) form if surgery is happening with shorter notice. The nursing staff will be responsible for ensuring administration is done in a timely manner can help reduce acute rejection in the first phase of post-transplant care.

The role of the floor nurse is very important to help ensure the success of the transplant. Because the organ transplant procedure is so delicate, there are many things that must be followed closely during initial postoperative care. There are indicators of decline that must be recognized and reported in a timely manner to practitioners and physicians to help promote healthy graft function. Pain over the surgical site, reduction in output, fever, or lab changes must be reported promptly. Having a specially trained registered nurse is preferred, and often the patient-to-nurse ratio is 1:1.

Immediate postoperative care for a kidney transplant is very extensive. There are multifaceted needs of the patient. Ensuring proper input and output will help the provider understand the quality of graft function, as well as the electrolyte and renal panels that will be drawn frequently. Timed labs are important as the patient labs will fluctuate greatly immediately postoperatively. IV fluids, as well as infection prevention medications, will be administered and in the treatment plan. Ensuring staff is monitoring vitals and temperature closely is imperative to catch postoperative complications and infections quickly. Medications are often time-sensitive, and staff must be timely with administration and educating patients about this. There will also be routine postoperative precautions for venous thromboembolism prophylaxis and pain management.

There are several complications that can occur with a major solid organ transplant such as a kidney transplant. Acute rejection is the most common, occurring in almost 1 in 3 patients. Acute rejection usually occurs within the first thirty days of transplant but can happen at any time. Close monitoring of drug levels, electrolytes, and renal function panels will be important. The caregiver post-surgery must also be comfortable with the acceptable ranges for a newly transplanted organ and know when to call and report concerns. Some of the immunosuppressant drugs used to prevent rejection can be nephrotoxic if dose is too high, such as cyclosporin or tacrolimus. On the contrary, if the drug level is not high enough, then the immune system can attack the new organ. Labs will be drawn daily to every other day for drug levels and renal panels to ensure avoiding nephrotoxicity as well as graft function.[14] On occasion, a patient may still need bicarbonate supplementation or potassium replacement. There are some cases where the graft function is delayed, and hemodialysis is also needed to help with fluid balance or electrolytes until graft is properly functioning. Taking this all into consideration the floor nursing staff must be prudent in assessment skills, multitasking, and know what is abnormal and what to report to the transplant team while the patient is hospitalized. The average hospitalization is 3 to 7 days after the procedure. Once discharged follow-up visits are frequent until deemed stable.

Although a superior treatment method for patients with ESRD, a transplant brings many risks and potential complications. Operative complications can occur, related to vascular, urologic, and parietal issues. Patient will be immunosuppressed the remainder of their life. There are increased incidences of opportunistic infections, cancer, and other medication side effects that are not desirable. Immediately posttransplant the patient is put on prophylactic medications for opportunistic infection. The three main causes of death after transplant are infection, cardiovascular disease, and cancer.[15] These items are high priority to prevent.

The highest cause of death noted in a posttransplant patient is an infection, accounting for 53% of all deaths.[15] In addition to the complex immunosuppression regimen after transplant patients are often prescribed antivirals and antibiotics to prevent this. Commonly, post-transplant patients are more prone to thrush, cytomegalovirus (CMV), and Pneumocystis pneumonia as well as other viral and other fungal infection. The risk is at an all-time high directly post-surgery as this is when the patient is most immunocompromised. CMV is the most commonly found opportunistic infection, occurring in approximately 8% of patients.[16] Bactrim is commonly the first choice to give patients to prevent pneumonia, as long as they are not allergic to sulfa.[17] Often the patient is prescribed a mouthwash rinse for thrush and to also prevent mouth sores. For CMV prophylaxis they are advised to be given oral ganciclovir or valganciclovir.[16] A patient also is prone to BK virus, a virus that can cause nephropathy, and Epstein–Barr virus, which may cause acute tubular necrosis or tubulointerstitial nephritis. The occurrence of BK polyomavirus nephropathy can be found in approximately 10% of kidney transplant recipients.[16] This new medication regimen of multiple immunosuppressants, steroids, and various preventative antibacterial and antivirals can be very confusing and difficult for the patient to adapt to as they often have other medications they also have to take.

Ensuring education to the patient about each drug being given and teaching them about the importance of consistency is important. Immunosuppressants have a lot of side effects that the patient must also learn how to manage. Some of the most common such as nausea, headaches, hyperglycemia, dyspnea, diarrhea, and abdominal pain occur in greater than 10% of the population prescribed these medications. Unfortunately, these can be symptoms renal patients are familiar with; however, even when they are undesirable the patient must understand the medications are very important to take regularly and communicate with the transplant team to find the best options to manage these. Without long-term immunosuppression, they compromise the health of the kidney as the body will go into rejection sometimes as soon as one missed dose.

Cardiovascular disease is tied closely with patients with ESRD. Hypertension being a major contributor to kidney function decline gives many patients who are coming in for transplants preexisting cardiovascular disease risk factors. Left ventricular hypertrophy and congestive heart failure commonly are comorbid conditions for patients with ESRD. Vascular complications of the patient with CKD also can occur due to things such as hypervolemia, anemia, and bone mineral disease.[18] Transplant surgery manipulates the aortic artery as this is where the organ is connected for perfusion. It is noted that vascular complications, such as thrombosis or stenosis of the renal artery or vein, or more rare complications such as aneurysms, arteriovenous fistulas, or hematoma are the most serious to correct once identified as they have a high incidence of graft dysfunction if they occur.[12] To prevent cardiovascular events, ensuring proper antihypertensive regimens, blood pressure monitoring, and cardiology follow-up is important.

Once a patient is discharged home, a transplant patient still has a long way to go with recovery. The complex medication regimen and close monitoring does not end. Patient is often expected to report to the transplant clinic twice a week for labs and assessment, the visits then taper off with frequency as time goes on. Medications will change frequently, based off drug levels or electrolyte panels. Patients are educated on safety with protecting the organ as it is placed in the lower pelvic region as opposed to the mid back where native kidneys are anatomically located. The rationale for this is that it is less invasive for surgery and is easier to monitor after surgery. Patents are often asked to give up contact sports and be cautious of strenuous activity that could increase the risk for herniation. The native kidneys are often left in place unless they are cancerous or have cysts that are causing pain or infection. Eventually, the native kidneys shrink in size to approximately the size of a walnut, unless the underlying renal failure was due to polycystic disease. Communicating with their primary care doctor and other health care professionals about their transplant is also important as often transplant recipients need to still avoid nonsteroidal anti-inflammatory drug, and often have to dose adjust medications such as antibiotics.

Patients are asked to follow a healthy lifestyle to adhere to a healthy balanced diet. They may still require a diabetic or cardiac diet, based on other comorbid conditions they have. Often patients have difficulty keeping up with the intake of fluids as they were limited on fluid intake so long on dialysis. On occasion, they are given outpatient IV fluids. Patients must relearn what is healthy and how to stick to proper portion sizes. Renal diet can limit sometimes even healthy foods due to potassium and phosphorous restrictions. Because a patient now is healthy, their appetite picks up. Steroid use after transplant will also contribute to increases appetite and patients often gain weight. To avoid obesity and steroid-induced diabetes they must work closely with a dietician and social worker. Exercise is also highly encouraged.

Maintaining insurance for medication cost, specialty providers, hospitalization and procedures is important. When a patient is on dialysis, they are able to be on Medicare before being 65 years old, and qualify for disability. Patients who transplant and are under 65 years old may have to consider going back to work. Medicare only covers up to 3 years posttransplant unless the patient is over 65 or eligible for another reason. To avoid lapse in insurance it is recommended to have two insurances to cover the transplant costs and avoid coverage loss once the 3-year mark after transplant. Without coverage immunosuppressives are very expensive.

The goal posttransplant is to have the patient return to as normal as a life as they can. Women of childbearing age can carry and have successful pregnancies. There is a International Transplant Pregnancy Registry that helps trend and follow these situations, and people worldwide with all types of organ transplants have had success. It is an ongoing research study that is tracking the effects of pregnancy on transplant recipients and the effects of immunosuppressive medications on fertility and pregnancy outcomes.[19] If a patient with a transplant chooses to try for pregnancy, the immunosuppression regimen changes as often the medications are dangerous to an unborn fetus and can lead to birth defects or miscarriage.

SUMMARY

As we have discussed, organ transplantation is the best option for patients to have a more normal life and the longest life expectancy. Having less people on dialysis also benefits the Medicare system by reducing costs of care. The care for these patients is complex and will require lifelong medication, screenings, and follow-up. All disciplines of health care play a role in the success of a major organ transplant surgery success. With expanding knowledge of this complex procedure to more health care workers there is hope that better care can be provided to optimize the lifespans of these valuable gifts. The reality of transplantation is that it is a medical treatment, not a cure. Many people who transplant will live long enough to have to return to dialysis or be re-listed for another transplant so keeping the graft healthy as long as possible is the ultimate goal.

CLINICS CARE POINTS

- Kidney transplantation is a treatment option for end stage renal disease patients, but is not a cure.
- The process for organ donation and matching is complex and requires multidisciplinary involvement.
- This treatment plan does not come without risk. There are intra-operative and post-operative complications that must be monitored and treated.

- A transplant recipient must be followed by a transplant nephrologist for the lifespan of the organ.
- Having awareness of common complications helps the care team provide best possible care.
- Transplantation brings less cost burden to Medicare.
- Patient involvement in education on medication therapy and importance of their own health management post-transplant will help prolong lifespan of the organ.

DISCLOSURE

The author has no financial or commercial conflicts of interest related to this project.

REFERENCES

1. Jack K-C, Philip K-T. Chronic kidney disease epidemic: how do we deal with it? Nephrology 2018;23(Suppl 4):116–20.
2. CDC and Department of Health and Human Services, Chronic kidney disease in United States. 2021. Available at: https://www.cdc.gov/kidneydisease/publications-resources/ckd-national-facts.html.
3. Center for Medicare and Medicaid Services, Medicare program; end-stage renal disease prospective payment system, Payment for renal dialysis services Furnished to Individuals with acute kidney injury, and end-stage renal disease quality incentive program. 2020. Available at: https://www.cms.gov/newsroom/fact-sheets/medicare-program-end-stage-renal-disease-prospective-payment-system-payment-renal-dialysis-services.
4. Elflien J. Donor designation rates in the U.S. in 2018, by state. 2018. Available at: https://www.statista.com/statistics/624834/state-designated-organ-donors-among-us-adults-by-state/.
5. NIH National Institute of Diabetes and Digestive and Kidney Diseases, Kidney disease statistics for the United States. 2021. Available at: https://www.niddk.nih.gov/health-information/health-statistics/kidneydisease.
6. NSH, Risks kidney transplant. 2021. Available at: https://www.nhs.uk/conditions/kidney- transplant/risks/.
7. KDIGO, Transplantation. Official J Transplant Soc Int Liver Soc, 104 (4s). 2020. Available at: https://kdigo.org/wp- content/uploads/2018/08/KDIGO-Txp-Candidate-GL-FINAL.pdf.
8. Health Resources and Service Administration (HRSA), Organ donation statistics. 2021. Available at: https://www.organdonor.gov/learn/organ-donation-statistics.
9. USRDS, Health expenditures with persons with ESRD, Annu Data Rep volume 2. 2020. Available at: https://adr.usrds.org/2020/end-stage-renal-disease/9-health care-expenditures-for-persons–esrd.
10. American Kidney Fund, Types of transplants. 2022. Available at: https://www.kidneyfund.org/kidney- disease/kidney-failure/treatment-of-kidney-failure/kidney-transplant/types-of-transplants/#living-donor-transplant.
11. Baker R, Mark P, Patel R, et al. Renal association clinical care practice guideline in postoperative care in the kidney transplant recipient. BMC Nephrol 2017; 18:174.
12. Reyna-Sepúlveda F, Ponce-Escobedo A, Guevara-Charles A, et al. Outcomes and surgical complications in kidney transplantation. Int J Organ Transpl Med 2017;8(2):78–84.

13. Emory Health care, Kidney transplant program: becoming a patient. 2021. Available at. emoryhealthcare.org.
14. Kasiske B, Zeier M, Chapman J, et al. KDIGO clinical practice guideline for the care of kidney transplant recipients: a summary. Kidney Int 2009;77(4):299–311.
15. Nefrol J. Understanding the causes of mortality post transplantation- There is more than meets the eye. Braz J Nephrol 2018;40(2):102–4.
16. Karuthu S, Blumburg E. Common infections in kidney transplant recipients. Clin J Am Soc Nephrol 2012;7(12):2058–70.
17. Fishman J, Alexander B. Prophylaxis of infections in solid organ transplant, Prophylaxis of infections in solid organ transplantation. UpToDate; 2020.
18. Birdwell K, Park M. Post-transplant cardiovascular disease. Clin J Am Soc Nephrol 2021;16(12):1878–89.
19. Transplant Pregnancy Registry, About the registry. 2022. Available at: https://www.transplantpregnancyregistry.org/.

Onco-Nephrology in the Critical Care Setting

Recognizing and Treating Renal Manifestations of Cancer and Oncological Emergencies

Kelli Frost, MS, PA-C

KEYWORDS

- Onco-nephrology • Tumor lysis syndrome • Hypercalcemia • Critical care nursing

KEY POINTS

- Onco-nephrology is an emerging subspecialty of nephrology and kidney-related oncological conditions are frequently seen in the critical care setting.
- Acute kidney injury and chronic kidney disease are common in patients with cancer and can impact their treatment course and long-term morbidity and mortality.
- Tumor lysis syndrome is a life-threatening oncological emergency that requires prompt recognition and treatment.
- Malignancy-associated hypercalcemia is a frequent complication of cancer that may present at any point throughout the course of disease.
- Critical care nurses plan an important role in the recognition and treatment of onco-nephrology conditions.

INTRODUCTION

The subspeciality of Onco-Nephrology is concerned with the care of patients with cancer and kidney disease. It is a relatively newer field of study that became formally recognized by the American Society of Nephrology in 2011 when it formed an Onco-Nephrology Forum Group.[1] Over the past ten years, Onco-Nephrology has grown rapidly and now includes increasing research activity, national conferences, journals, consult services, and fellowship programs.[2,3] This path led to the development of the American Society of Onco-Nephrology in 2022, whose mission is to provide a forum for idea exchange and education.[4] The emerging discipline of Onco-Nephrology sits at the intersection of oncology and nephrology, studying both the acute and chronic renal manifestations due to malignancy or its treatment (**Table 1**).[5] These conditions include obstructive nephropathy, electrolyte disorders,

University of Detroit Mercy, 4001 West McNichols Road, Detroit, MI 48221, USA
E-mail address: battankl@udmercy.edu

Crit Care Nurs Clin N Am 34 (2022) 453–466
https://doi.org/10.1016/j.cnc.2022.07.002
0899-5885/22/© 2022 Elsevier Inc. All rights reserved.

Table 1
Renal manifestation of cancer by type

Cancer Type	Renal Manifestation
All cancers	AKI from drug toxicity
Leukemia	Drug toxicity AKI from sepsis (ATN) Prerenal AKI due to volume depletion AKI due to TLS
Myeloma	AKI from volume depletion Myeloma kidney
Lymphoma	AKI due to TLS
Renal cell carcinoma	Obstructive uropathy Drug toxicity Nephrectomy resulting in CKD
Lung	Toxicity due to platinum-based chemotherapy
GI and GYN	Obstructive uropathy

Abbreviations: AKI, acute kidney injury; ATN, acute tubular necrosis; CKD, chronic kidney disease; TLS, tumor lysis syndrome.
Data from Abudayyeh AA, Lahoti A, Salahudeen AK. Onconephrology: The need and the emergence of a subspecialty in nephrology. Kidney Int. 2014;85(5):1002-4.

acute kidney injury (AKI), and tumor lysis syndrome (TLS).[6] A multitude of other Onco-Nephrology topics are vital to the specialty but are beyond the scope of this publication. This article explores the general concepts of renal disease in malignancy and the acute oncological emergencies of TLS and hypercalcemia that may be seen in the critical care setting. Optimal care of patients with cancer and renal abnormalities requires a multidisciplinary collaboration between oncology, nephrology, urology, critical care, pharmacy, nursing, and palliative care to increase the cancer cure rate and survival time.[7,8] These Onco-Nephrology partnerships will also foster ongoing research and guideline development to outline the best practices in caring for cancer patients with kidney disease.

DISCUSSION

Chronic kidney disease (CKD) is common in patients with cancer, estimated to range from 40% having stage 2 CKD to 2% having stage 5 CKD.[7] The presence of CKD impacts medication dosing and increases the risk for potential side effects of treatment. Since the kidneys are the elimination pathway for many oncology drugs, dose adjustment may be required, which may lead to inadequate dosing and poor treatment outcomes.[9] CKD following cancer treatment may be due to nephrectomy and chemotherapy toxicities.

Patients with baseline normal renal function can develop AKI from their underlying malignancy or the medications used to treat the disease. A large Denmark study found the 1-year risk of AKI in patients with cancer was 17.5%, with the 5-year risk being as high as 27%.[10] In the critical care setting, renal failure due to AKI is prevalent in up to 50% of patients with underlying malignancy.[11] The risk for AKI is higher in critically ill patients with cancer as compared to other critically ill patients. Data in the last 10 years has? revealed a link between renal insufficiency and reduced overall survival and increased cancer-related mortality.[12] AKI in critically ill patients can cause pauses or interruptions in cancer therapy, and increase the duration of ventilator support, length of stay, cost, morbidity, and mortality.[13,14] The significant renal dysfunction seen in critically ill patients may require renal replacement therapy, which is associated with a 72% to 85% mortality rate.[15]

AKI is often multifactorial in the critically ill patient. Causes that are similar to other intensive care patients include sepsis, shock, and non-oncology medications such as nonsteroidal anti-inflammatory drugs and ACE inhibitors. Laboratory indicators of renal failure include low urine volume, elevated serum blood urea nitrogen (BUN) or creatinine (CR), and hyperkalemia.[13] AKI due to malignancy can be classified into prerenal, intrinsic, and postrenal causes. Prerenal causes include chemotherapy-induced nausea, vomiting, and diarrhea that lead to volume depletion, sepsis, hypercalcemia, or impaired cardiac output. Prerenal kidney failure may present with oliguria, tachycardia, and hypotension.[13] Additional physical exam findings are dependent on the cause of the prerenal kidney failure. Intrinsic kidney injury can result from acute tubular necrosis or acute interstitial nephritis because of cancer treatment, cast nephropathy, antibiotics, intravenous contrast dye, and sepsis. Most chemotherapy agents, including targeted therapy and immunotherapy, have the potential to cause intrinsic kidney injury. Postrenal AKI causes include urinary outlet obstruction associated with bladder, prostate, or gynecological tumors, or deposition of uric acid crystals in the renal tubules as seen with TLS.[9,11,16]

Tumor lysis syndrome

TLS is an oncological emergency characterized by hyperuricemia, hyperkalemia, hyperphosphatemia, hypocalcemia, and AKI. This dangerous condition develops when tumor cells lyse and release their intracellular materials into circulation. The body cannot compensate for the rapid influx of potassium, phosphorus, and nucleic acids, and subsequent electrolyte imbalances and AKI may develop (**Fig. 1**). TLS can occur spontaneously or more commonly after treatment with chemotherapy, radiation, or corticosteroids.[17] The laboratory abnormalities due to TLS are typically seen at 6 h to 7 days after treatment but can occur weeks after treatment. Although TLS can occur at any point during that period, patients are at the greatest risk during the first 6–48 h after treatment. TLS can affect the neurological, cardiac, gastrointestinal, and muscular systems. The general clinical manifestations of TLS are nausea, vomiting, lethargy, edema, fluid overload, and muscle cramps, with the most severe manifestations being cardiac arrhythmias and seizures.[18] If TLS is not recognized and treated quickly and adequately, death will result in up to 50% of patients.[19]

Cancer types most likely to develop TLS have rapid cell turnover and increased sensitivity to therapy. These include high-grade lymphoma, acute myeloid leukemia, small-cell lung cancer, and germ cell tumors.[18] Malignancy types can be categorized by their risk for the development of TLS (**Table 2**). TLS is rarely seen in patients with solid tumors, but it is thought the true incidence is underreported due to lower index of suspicion and reporting in this patient population. Interestingly, the TLS mortality rate was found to be higher in that same group of patients because of lower rates of prophylaxis and awareness of the complication.[20] The life-threatening TLS is being increasingly seen after treatment with novel targeted therapies and immunotherapy, with case reports of TLS in patients receiving monoclonal antibodies, tyrosine kinase inhibitors, proteasome inhibitors, and immunomodulatory agents.[21–24] In fact, any treatment that is an effective therapy for cancer and causes lysis of malignant cells can potentially lead to TLS.[25] Patient-specific risk factors for TLS include high tumor burden, advanced age, male sex, lactate dehydrogenase greater than two times the upper limit of normal, white blood cell count greater than 50×10^9/L, extensive

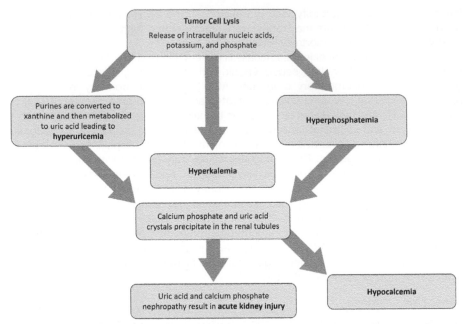

Fig. 1. Pathophysiology of tumor lysis syndrome. (*Data from* Rosner MH, Perazella MA, Lerma EV. *CURRENT diagnosis & treatment: Nephrology & hypertension.* 2nd ed. New York, NY: McGraw-Hill Education LLC; 2018.)

metastases, bone marrow involvement, underlying CKD, pretreatment hyperuricemia, and dehydration.[26,27]

TLS can be classified as laboratory or clinical. Laboratory TLS is defined as two or more abnormalities in uric acid, potassium, or phosphorus levels within 3 days before or up to 7 days after treatment (**Table 3**).[18] Clinical TLS includes the laboratory

Table 2 Risk for tumor lysis syndrome	
High risk	High-grade non-Hodgkin lymphoma (Burkitt lymphoma) Lymphoblastic lymphoma Mantle cell lymphoma (bulky disease) Acute myeloid leukemia with high-risk features Acute lymphoblastic leukemia
Intermediate risk	Acute myeloid leukemia with low-risk features Small-cell lung carcinoma Germ cell tumor Low-grade non-Hodgkin lymphoma Chronic lymphocytic leukemia treated with targeted therapy
Low risk	Most solid tumors Chronic myeloid leukemia in the chronic phase Myeloma

Data from Darmon M, Ciroldi M, Thiery G, Schlemmer B, Azoulay E. Clinical review: Specific aspects of acute renal failure in cancer patients. *Critical Care (London, England).* 2006:10(2):211 and Cairo MS, Bishop M. Tumor lysis syndrome: New therapeutic strategies and classification. *British Journal of haematology.* 2004; 127(1):3-11.

Table 3		
Cairo-Bishop definition of laboratory and clinical tumor lysis syndrome		
		Diagnostic Criteria
Laboratory TLS	Potassium	$\geq$ 6 mEq/L or 25% increase from baseline
	Phosphorus	$\geq$ 4.5 mEq/L or 25% increase from baseline
	Uric acid	$\geq$ 8 mEq/L or 25% increase from baseline
	Calicum	25% decrease from baseline
Clinical TLS	Laboratory TLS, plus one or more of the following: • Acute kidney injury (serum creatinine $\geq$ 1.5 times ULN) • Seizure • Cardiac arrhythmia or sudden death	

Abbreviations: TLS, tumor lysis syndrome; ULN, upper limit normal.

Data from Cairo MS, Bishop M, Tumor lysis syndrome: New therapeutic strategies and classification. *British journal of haematology.* 2004; 127(1):3-11.

abnormalities plus the presence of seizure, arrhythmias, or AKI. Only a small percentage of patients with laboratory TLS will develop clinical TLS. Patients with clinical TLS have a higher risk of mortality.[28] TLS can also be graded from 1 to 5 to define the severity of the condition. Cairo and Bishop described a grading system based on the level of Cr elevation, the presence and type of cardiac arrhythmia, and the presence of and severity of seizures.[28]

Potassium is primarily stored in the intracellular space. Hyperkalemia develops when malignant cells lyse and release high levels of potassium into the extracellular space. It is typically the first electrolyte abnormality in TLS.[29] Symptoms of hyperkalemia include nausea, vomiting, diarrhea, anorexia, lethargy, muscle weakness, cramps, and paresthesias.[18] Hyperkalemia is often considered the most dangerous consequence of TLS due to its impact on the cardiac system and risk of sudden death.[30] Electrocardiographic (EKG) changes seen in hyperkalemia include prolonged PR interval, arrhythmia, widened QRS, peaked T waves, and asystole.[17]

Malignant cells contain higher levels of intracellular phosphorus than nonmalignant cells.[26] When phosphorus binds to calcium, an insoluble calcium-phosphate crystal is formed. These crystals can precipitate in the kidneys through a process called nephrocalcinosis, which causes AKI. Patients with hyperphosphatemia may complain of muscle cramping or present with tetany and seizure.

When tumor cells break open, their nucleic acids spill into the extracellular space. The nucleic acids are converted to hypoxanthine and then xanthine, followed by conversion to uric acid. In other mammals, uric acid can be processed further to allantoin by urate oxidase. Humans lack this enzyme and uric acid circulates in the extracellular space before being excreted by the kidneys in the urine.[28] During TLS, the increased levels of uric acid overwhelm the kidney's capacity for excretion. Hyperuricemia usually develops 48–72 h after treatment begins.[31] The uric acid then crystallizes in the renal tubules and causes an obstructive nephropathy. An additional mechanism of injury caused by uric acid crystals is cytokine-induced inflammation.

Hypocalcemia is the result of high levels of circulating phosphorus binding to calcium to form calcium phosphate crystals. It can manifest as muscle cramps, tetany, hypotension, arrhythmias, and seizures. Severe hypocalcemia can result in cardiac failure, coma, and death. In most cases, calcium should not be replaced until there is significant cardiovascular or neurovascular complications. Calcium supplementation in the setting of acute hyperphosphatemia will promote further development and deposition of calciumphosphate crystals.

AKI during TLS results primarily from precipitation of uric acid crystals and deposition of calcium phosphate crystals in the renal tubules.[21] Additional mechanisms of renal injury because of elevated uric acid are renal vasoconstriction and pro-inflammatory effects.[32,33] The resulting AKI can be mild or severe enough to cause oliguria and uremia. Clinical manifestations include nausea, vomiting, lethargy, edema, hypertension, electrolyte disturbances, and acidosis. Other multifactorial contributors to AKI in the critical care setting are nephrotoxic drugs, dehydration, and sepsis. A high anion gap metabolic acidosis leads to decreased intracellular uptake of potassium and uric acid solubility and a shift of phosphorus into the extracellular space, further worsening the electrolyte disturbances.[21] TLS with AKI is a poor prognostic factor and is associated with increased short-term and long-term mortality and risk for subsequent CKD.[34]

Therapeutic options

It is vitally important to monitor for and immediately treat TLS because patients with clinical TLS have an increased risk of morbidity and mortality.[9] The most important approach is prevention and maintaining a high index of suspicion for the development of laboratory and clinical TLS. Patients are first risk-stratified to determine the treatment plan. Low-risk patients can be volume expanded orally and monitored for fluid status and laboratory abnormalities, whereas intermediate-risk patients should be started on IV hydration and oral allopurinol.[35] Before treatment, high-risk patients should be identified and prophylactically started on IV hydration and either allopurinol or rasburicase. Allopurinol is a competitive inhibitor of xanthine oxidase and prevents the metabolism of xanthine and hypoxanthine to uric acid. This will decrease the formation of new uric acid.[18] Rasburicase is a recombinant urate oxidase that functions to convert uric acid into allantoin. Unlike uric acid, allantoin is easily excreted in the urine. If a patient is at high risk for TLS, cancer treatment may need to be delayed allowing for prophylaxis. The choice of allopurinol or rasburicase for prophylaxis is based on the tumor and patient risk factors for TLS. The practice of administering sodium bicarbonate for urine alkalization before cancer treatment is no longer universally recommended.[28] Urinary alkalization does increase uric acid solubility and excretion, but at the expense of potentially increasing the renal crystallization and deposition of xanthine, hypoxanthine, and calcium phosphate.[36]

Despite prophylactic measures, up to 5% of patients will develop laboratory and/or clinical TLS.[37] In patients who develop TLS during or after cancer treatment, the mainstay of care in TLS is aggressive hydration and rapid correction of electrolyte disturbances and hyperuricemia (**Table 4**). High urine output will promote excretion of uric acid and phosphorus. The patient should be given 0.9 normal saline at a rate to maintain a urine output of 100 to 200 milliliters per hour. Fluid balance should be monitored closely in patients with oliguric renal failure and heart failure. Allopurinol is not indicated in the treatment of acute TLS because it does not eliminate the uric acid already present in circulation. In addition, blocking the conversion of xanthine and hypoxanthine to uric acid will increase the circulating levels of those precursors and promote further obstructive nephropathy. Rasburicase is the treatment of choice in acute laboratory or clinical TLS to promote elimination of uric acid. Renal and hepatic dose adjustments are not required.[38] The drug is a safe, yet expensive, method to quickly reduce the uric acid level. Potential side effects of rasburicase include anaphylaxis in less than 1% of patients, and more commonly gastrointestinal symptoms, fever, and headache.[39] One contradiction to rasburicase is use in patients with glucose-6-phosphate dehydrogenase deficiency. In this patient population, the uric acid

Table 4
Treatment of laboratory and clinical tumor lysis syndrome

	Treatment
General	Aggressive IV hydration to maintain urine output of 100–200 mL/h Electrolyte monitoring every 6–12 h Continuous EKG monitoring Avoid nephrotoxic agents Dialysis when indicated
Hyperuricemia	Allopurinol: IV or oral dosing based on creatinine clearance Rasburicase
Hyperkalemia	Sodium polystyrene sulfonate orally Inhaled beta-agonists IV insulin and dextrose IV calcium gluconate if EKG changes Sodium bicarbonate IV if acidosis Dietary restriction of potassium Eliminate IV or oral potassium sources Eliminate mediations that may increase potassium levels
Hyperphosphatemia	Oral phosphate binders Dietary restriction of phosphate
Hypocalcemia	Monitor calcium level if asymptomatic IV calcium gluconate with EKG monitoring if symptomatic

Abbreviations: EKG, electrocardiograph; IV, intravenous.
Data from McGraw, Beth, RN, BSN, OCN. At an increased risk: Tumor lysis syndrome. Clin J oncol Nurs. 2008; 12(4): 563-5 and Muslimani A, Chisti MM, Wills S, et al. How we treat tumor lysis syndrome. Oncology (Williston Park, N Y). 2011; 25(4):369-375.

breakdown byproduct hydrogen peroxide cannot be metabolized and causes severe hemolysis.[40]

Hyperkalemia associated with TLS is treated by shifting potassium back into the intracellular space and promoting potassium excretion through the kidneys and gastrointestinal tract. The fastest way to shift potassium into the intracellular space and lower serum potassium is by treatment with inhaled beta-agonist and intravenous insulin and glucose. Adding sodium polystyrene will promote potassium exchange across the gastrointestinal mucosa.[17] An important step in the management of hyperkalemia is a medication review, noting medications that may impair tubular secretion of potassium such as angiotension-converting enzyme inhibitors and potassium-sparing diuretics.[41] Hyperphosphatemia is treated with oral phosphate binders such as aluminum hydroxide. Symptomatic hypocalcemia can be replaced with intravenous calcium gluconate. Renal replacement therapy is recommended when hydration and optimal pharmacological treatments fail to adequately correct the severe laboratory abnormalities, or if uremia, volume overload, uncontrolled hypertension, or acidosis develop.[18,28]

Malignancy-associated hypercalcemia

Hypercalcemia is defined as a serum calcium level greater than 10.5 mg per dL or an ionized calcium level greater than 5.6 mg per dL. Ionized calcium is the best marker for hypercalcemia since serum calcium is a poor indicator of total body calcium due to albumin binding. The rate of calcium increase is often more important for symptom development and severity than the absolute calcium level.[42] Most patients with mild hypercalcemia will be asymptomatic and the elevated calcium level will be an incidental finding on routine labs. When hypercalcemia becomes symptomatic, the complaints can be nonspecific and include muscle cramping, constipation, anorexia, weakness, fatigue, nausea, and vomiting (**Box 1**).[43,44] Many times these vague complaints are overlooked or attributed to treatment side effects or other chronic medical conditions. Neurological symptoms such as mental status changes and coma are most often seen with severe hypercalcemia, along with complications of renal tubular acidosis, nephrolithiasis, acute or chronic renal failure, bradycardia, hypotension, and arrhythmia. Hypercalcemia can often lead to nephrogenic diabetes insipidus and severe volume depletion due to polyuria.[26] This combined with nausea, vomiting, and anorexia often leads to significant dehydration, which can worsen hypercalcemia and result in prerenal AKI.

Malignancy-associated hypercalcemia (MAH) is a frequent complication of cancer, occurring in 20% to 30% of patients at some point throughout the course of their disease.[11,17] It can present at any point during the spectrum of a patient's cancer journey, potentially as an acute emergency. In some patients, the hypercalcemia precedes the cancer diagnosis and is the first presenting manifestation of malignancy.[45] Hypercalcemia in patients with cancer is caused by one of three mechanisms. Humoral MAH is a paraneoplastic process and is seen in up to 80% of cases of hypercalcemia of malignancy. In humoral MAH, parathyroid hormone-related protein (PTHrP) is secreted by malignant cells and stimulates osteoclast action in the bone and promotes increased calcium absorption in the kidney.[42,46] Solid tumors are most often associated with humoral MAH, including squamous cell carcinoma, adenocarcinoma, hepatocellular carcinoma, and cholangiocarcinoma. The second most common mechanism and seen in 20% of cases of MAH, is hypercalcemia associated with metastatic bone lesions. When metastatic lesions are found in the bone, most often seen in breast, lung, and kidney malignancies, there is osteolytic release of calcium from the bone and a subsequent increase in serum calcium levels.[26] The least common mechanism, seen in less than 1% of MAH, is mediated by calcitriol production. It should be noted that many instances of MAH are multifactorial. Unfortunately, MAH is a negative prognostic marker and median survival is less than 35 days after presentation.[47] The malignancy

---

Box 1
Symptoms of hypercalcemia

Nausea and vomiting

Anorexia

Abdominal pain

Constipation

Irritability and anxiety

Confusion, depression, lethargy, coma

Polyuria and nocturia and polydipsia

Dehydration

Fatigue

Muscle aches and weakness

Bradycardia

Data from Rosner MH, Perazella MA, Lerma EV. *CURRENT diagnosis & treatment: Nephrology & hypertension.* 2nd ed. New York, N Y: McGraw-Hill Education LLC; 2018.

types most associated with MAH are breast, lung, esophagus, and renal cell carcinomas, myeloma, and T-cell leukemia/lymphoma.[48]

Therapeutic options
The main goals of hypercalcemia treatment are aggressive hydration to correct dehydration, increasing renal excretion of calcium, inhibiting bone resorption of calcium, and treatment of the underlying malignancy (**Box 2**). Hydration will increase intravascular fluid volume, dilute the extracellular calcium concentration, and promote urinary excretion of excess calcium. Intravenous fluids should be given at a rate of 250 to 500 mL per hour until euvolemia is achieved and then 100 to 150 mL per hour to maintain a goal urine output of 100 to 150 mL per hour.[14,49,50] The IV fluid of choice is 0.9 normal saline. Loop diuretics can be cautiously added in cases where fluid overload develops. Thiazide diuretics should be avoided entirely as they stimulate renal calcium reabsorption.[48] In addition, IV phosphate should be avoided as this may promote nephrocalcinosis because of calcium-phosphate binding and deposition in the kidney.

Bisphosphonates are used to treat hypercalcemia of malignancy. Bisphosphonates work by reducing osteoclast activity and promoting osteoclast apoptosis.[26] Options for bisphosphonate treatment are zoledronic acid and pamidronate. Both medications show adequate and similar calcium-lowering rate.[51] Pamidronate is preferred in patients with renal insufficiency and Cr clearance of less than 30 milliliters per minute. Bisphosphonates have an onset of action of 48 to 72 h and can have a persistent effect for up to one month. The bisphosphonates are generally well tolerated, and side effects include bone pain, fever, chills, osteonecrosis of the jaw, and possible atrial fibrillation.[52,53] When more immediate calcium lowering is needed, calcitonin can be used in the short term to quickly reduce calcium levels. Calcitonin works by inhibiting bone resorption and increasing calcium excretion in the urine. Adequate dosing will result in lowered serum calcium within 6–12 h. This effect is short-lived due to tachyphylaxis and dosing beyond 48 h is not recommended.[46] Glucocorticoids are an additional option in patients with hypercalcemia due to overproduction of calcitriol or in patient that are unable to receive bisphosphonates due to severe AKI. In cases of treatment failure, severe fluid overload, or life-threatening hypercalcemia, hemodialysis is a treatment option. It is important to understand that hypercalcemia of malignancy will

---

Box 2
Treatment options for hypercalcemia of malignancy

Hydration with 0.9 normal saline to goal urine output of 100–150 mL per hour

Discontinue calcium supplementation and thiazide diuretics

Bisphosphonates treatment with pamidronate or zoledronic acid

Calcitonin for rapid reduction of calcium levels

Glucocorticoids for hypercalcemia in lymphoma

Hemodialysis for severe symptomatic or refractory hypercalcemia

Treatment of underlying malignancy

Data from Rosner MH, Perazella MA, Lerma EV. *CURRENT diagnosis & treatment: Nephrology & hypertension.* 2nd ed. New York, N Y: McGraw-Hill Education LLC; 2018 and Jafari A, Rezaei-Tavirani M, Salimi M, Tavakkol R, Jafari Z. Oncological emergencies from pathophysiology and diagnosis to treatment: A narrative review. *Social work in public health.* 2020;35(8): 689-709.

recur without treatment of the underlying cancer and patients should be educated on the expected course of the disease.

SUMMARY

Patients with cancer account for 14% to 22% of admissions to the intensive care setting and require individualized care due to their complex diagnoses and multitude of potential oncology treatments.[54] Critical care nurses should have a baseline knowledge of cancer types and be familiar with the life-threatening conditions that may present at any point in the care of oncology patients, from initial onset to end-stage. Oncological emergencies such as TLS and MAH require prompt recognition and treatment and this knowledge will assist the critical care nurse in recognizing these oncology complications and reducing morbidity and mortality.[55]

All critically ill patients with cancer at risk for AKI should be monitored for contrast nephropathy and have their medications reviewed for potential elimination of nephrotoxic drugs. In patients at risk for or with the development of acute TLS or hypercalcemia, critical care nurses play an important role in management. Critical care nurses should be knowledgeable of the risk factors, laboratory abnormalities, and clinical manifestations of TLS and MAH in oncology patients undergoing cancer treatment.[56] Patient vitals should be monitored closely and continuous EKG monitoring for changes such as widened QRS, peaked T waves, and prolonged PR interval is required. Any indication of EKG changes should immediately be brought to the attention of the intensivist team caring for the patient. A thorough medication review should be done for all patients to identify medications that may worsen electrolyte disturbances and all IV fluids containing potassium, phosphorus, or calcium should be discontinued. If the patient develops AKI, all medications that are renally excreted should be dose modified for the level of renal impairment. The inputs, outputs, and patient weights should be frequently and accurately tracked and recorded to avoid fluid overload, especially in elderly patients or those with underlying CKD. Serial electrolyte monitoring should be performed every 6–12 h during the prophylaxis for and treatment of TLS.[18] In patients with mild to moderate hypercalcemia, there should be frequent mental status assessments to detect changes in cognition caused by increasing calcium levels.[43] Patients with mental status changes due to hypercalcemia should be closely monitored for wandering and falls.[57] Critical care nurses also play a role in ensuring that all exogenous calcium is removed from parental and enteral nutrition sources in patient with hypercalcemia.

Patients with AKI, TLS, and MAH have a poorer long-term prognosis and increased risk for morbidity and mortality. The critical care nurse is a valuable member of the treatment team during active treatment or end-of-life care and can encourage Palliative Care consultations earlier in the hospital stay to assist with treatment planning and goals of care discussions. Even in patients that are terminally ill, managing electrolyte disturbances can treat acute symptoms and improve quality of life. Critical care nurses, along with intensivists and oncologists, have an important role in education of the patient and their family throughout the course of care.

CLINICS CARE POINTS

- Patients with cancer with renal manifestations are frequently seen in the critical care setting.
- Acute kidney injury and oncological emergencies require prompt recognition and treatment.
- Tumor lysis syndrome is characterized by hyperkalemia, hyperphosphatemia, hyperuricemia, hypocalcemia, and acute kidney injury.

- Malignancy-associated hypercalcemia may manifest with vague complaints that can be overlooked or mistakenly attributed to cancer treatment.
- The primary treatment for both tumor lysis syndrome and malignancy-associated hypercalcemia is aggressive hydration.
- Allopurinol and rasburicase are used for the prevention and treatment of tumor lysis syndrome.
- Bisphosphonates are the treatment of choice for malignancy-associated hypercalcemia.
- Critical care patients with renal manifestations of malignancy require individualized care that includes frequent vitals and laboratory monitoring, strict input and output documentation, thorough medication review, and ongoing patient and family education.

DISCLOSURES

The author received no financial support for this article. The author has no potential conflict of interest with respect to the authorship or publication of this article.

REFERENCES

1. Thakkar J, Wanchoo R, Jhaveri KD. Onconephrology abstracts and publication trends: time to collaborate. Clin Kidney J 2015;8(5):629–31. Available at: https://www.ncbi.nlm.nih.gov/pubmed/26413292.
2. Rashidi A, Jhaveri KD, Workeneh BT, et al. The path toward the creation of the american society of onco-nephrology (ASON). J Onco-Nephrology 2022. https://doi.org/10.1177/23993693221079647. 23993693221079647.Available at:.
3. Journal of onco-nephrology. Available at: https://journals.sagepub.com/home/jnp Web site. Accessed March 10, 2022.
4. American society of onco-nephrology. Available at: www.ason-online.org. Accessed March 7, 2022.
5. Abudayyeh AA, Lahoti A, Salahudeen AK. Onconephrology: the need and the emergence of a subspecialty in nephrology. Kidney Int 2014;85(5):1002–4. Available at: https://ezproxy.libraries.udmercy.edu/login?url=https://www.proquest.com/scholarly-journals/onconephrology-need-emergence-subspecialty/docview/1520134748/se-2.
6. Jhaveri KD, Agarwal S. Onconephrology, an extra year of training: where do we stand? J Onco-Nephrology 2021;5(1):39–41.
7. Li Cavoli G, Rondello G, Li Cavoli T, et al. The onconephrology: our experience in patients with cancer. Saudi J Kidney Dis Transplant 2016;27(4):823–4.
8. Perazella MA. The kidney–cancer connection continues to grow. J Onco-Nephrology 2020;4(1–2):26–7. https://doi.org/10.1177/2399369320916474. Available at:.
9. Abudayyeh A. Onconephrology: an evolving field. Methodist DeBakey Cardiovasc J 2019;15(4):305–7.
10. Christiansen CF, Johansen MB, Langeberg WJ, et al. Incidence of acute kidney injury in patients with cancer : a Danish population-based cohort study. Eur J Intern Med 2011;22(4):399–406. Available at: https://www.clinicalkey.es/playcontent/1-s2.0-S0953620511000975.
11. Lam AQ, Humphreys BD. Onco-nephrology: AKI in the cancer patient. Clin J Am Soc Nephrol 2012;7(10):1692–700. http://cjasn.asnjournals.org/content/7/10/1692.abstract.

12. Launay-Vacher V, Porta C, Cosmai L. Introduction to the journal of onco-nephrology. J Onco-Nephrology 2017;1(1):1–4. https://journals.sagepub.com/doi/full/10.5301/jo-n.5000000.
13. Cooper D. Chapter 7: monitoring for renal dysfunction. In: Booker KJ, editor. Critical care nursing: monitoring and treatment of advanced nursing practice. Ames, IA: John Wiley & Sons; 2015. p. 380–402.
14. Routt M, Parks L. Critical care nursing of the oncology patient. 1st ed. Pittsburgh: Oncology Nursing Society; 2018. Available at: http://portal.igpublish.com/iglibrary/search/ONSB0000098.html.
15. Darmon M, Ciroldi M, Thiery G, et al. Clinical review: specific aspects of acute renal failure in patients with cancer. Crit Care (London, England) 2006;10(2):211. Available at: https://www-ncbi-nlm-nih-gov.ezproxy.libraries.udmercy.edu/pubmed/16677413.
16. HUMPHREYS BD, SOIFFER RJ, MAGEE CC. Renal failure associated with cancer and its treatment: an update. J Am Soc Nephrol 2005;16(1):151–61. Available at: https://www-ncbi-nlm-nih-gov.ezproxy.libraries.udmercy.edu/pubmed/15574506.
17. Oropello JM, Pastores SM, Kvetan V. Critical care. New York, NY: McGraw Hill; 2017.
18. Cairo MS, Bishop M. Tumour lysis syndrome: new therapeutic strategies and classification. Br J Haematol 2004;127(1):3–11. Available at: https://onlinelibrary.wiley.com/doi/abs/10.1111/j.1365-2141.2004.05094.x.
19. Coiffier B. Acute tumor lysis syndrome – a rare complication in the treatment of solid tumors. Oncol Res Treat 2010;33(10):498–9. Available at: https://www.karger.com/Article/Abstract/320581.
20. Baeksgaard L, Sørensen JB. Acute tumor lysis syndrome in solid tumors—a case report and review of the literature. Cancer Chemother Pharmacol 2003;51(3):187–92. Available at: https://www.ncbi.nlm.nih.gov/pubmed/12655435.
21. Muslimani A, Chisti MM, Wills S, et al. How we treat tumor lysis syndrome. Oncology (Williston Park, N.Y.) 2011;25(4):369–75. Available at: https://www.ncbi.nlm.nih.gov/pubmed/21618960.
22. Williams SM, Killeen AA. Tumor lysis syndrome. Arch Pathol Lab Med 2019;143(3):386–93. Available at: https://search.ebscohost.com/login.aspx?direct=true&db=ccm&AN=135037022&site=ehost-live.
23. Howard SC, Trifilio S, Gregory TK, et al. Tumor lysis syndrome in the era of novel and targeted agents in patients with hematologic malignancies: a systematic review. Ann Hematol 2016;95(4):563–73. Available at: https://link.springer.com/article/10.1007/s00277-015-2585-7.
24. Matuszkiewicz-Rowinska J, Malyszko J. Prevention and treatment of tumor lysis syndrome in the era of onco-nephrology progress. Kidney Blood Press Res 2020;45(5):645–60. Available at: https://www.karger.com/Article/FullText/509934.
25. Bose P, Qubaiah O. A review of tumour lysis syndrome with targeted therapies and the role of rasburicase. J Clin Pharm Ther 2011;36(3):299–326. Available at: https://api.istex.fr/ark:/67375/WNG-58RVL78P-S/fulltext.pdf.
26. Rosner MH, Perazella MA, Lerma EV. CURRENT diagnosis & treatment: nephrology & hypertension. 2nd ed. New York, N.Y: McGraw-Hill Education LLC; 2018. Available at: https://accessmedicine.mhmedical.com/book.aspx?bookid=2287.
27. Wilson FP, Berns JS. Onco-nephrology: tumor lysis syndrome. Clin J Am Soc Nephrol 2012;7(10):1730–9. Available at: http://cjasn.asnjournals.org/content/7/10/1730.abstract.

28. Coiffier B, Altman A, Pui C, et al. Guidelines for the management of pediatric and adult tumor lysis syndrome: an evidence-based review. J Clin Oncol 2008;26(16): 2767–78. Available at: http://jco.ascopubs.org/content/26/16/2767.abstract.
29. McGraw, Beth RN, BSN OCN. At an increased risk: tumor lysis syndrome. Clin J Oncol Nurs 2008;12(4):563–5. Available at: https://ezproxy.libraries.udmercy.edu/login?url=https://www.proquest.com/scholarly-journals/at-increased-risk-tumor-lysis-syndrome/docview/222743012/se-2?accountid=28018.
30. Howard SC, Jones DP, Pui C. The tumor lysis syndrome. N Engl J Med 2011; 364(19):1844–54,   10.1056/NEJMra0904569.   doi: 10.1056/NEJMra 0904569 Available at:.
31. Davidson MB, Thakkar S, Hix JK, et al. Pathophysiology, clinical consequences, and treatment of tumor lysis syndrome. Am J Med 2004;116(8):546–54.
32. Shimada M, Johnson RJ, May WS, et al. A novel role for uric acid in acute kidney injury associated with tumour lysis syndrome. Nephrol Dial Transplant 2009;24(10): 2960–4. Available at: https://api.istex.fr/ark:/67375/HXZ-GBBN18QD-R/fulltext.pdf.
33. Abdel-Nabey M, Chaba A, Serre J, et al. Tumor lysis syndrome, acute kidney injury and disease-free survival in critically ill patients requiring urgent chemotherapy. Ann Intensive Care 2022;12(1):15. Available at: https://link.springer.com/article/10.1186/s13613-022-00990-1.
34. Darmon M, Guichard I, Vincent F, et al. Prognostic significance of acute renal injury in acute tumor lysis syndrome. Leuk Lymphoma 2010;51(2):221–7. Available at: https://www.tandfonline.com/doi/abs/10.3109/10428190903456959.
35. Abousaud MI, Rush MC, Rockey M. Assessment of rasburicase utilization for tumor lysis syndrome management in pediatric and adult patients in the inpatient and outpatient settings. J Oncol Pharm Pract 2021;27(5):1165–71. Available at: https://journals.sagepub.com/doi/full/10.1177/1078155220945368.
36. Jameson JL, Kasper DL, Longo DL, et al. Harrison's principles of internal medicine. 20th edition. New York ; Chicago ; San Francisco: McGraw Hill Education; 2018.
37. Sarno J. Prevention and management of tumor lysis syndrome in adults with malignancy. J Adv Pract Oncol 2013;4(2):101–6. Available at: https://www.ncbi.nlm.nih.gov/pubmed/25031988.
38. Mayne N, Keady S, Thacker M. Rasburicase in the prevention and treatment of tumour lysis syndrome. Intensive Crit Care Nurs 2008;24(1):59–62. Available at: https://ezproxy.libraries.udmercy.edu/login?url=https://www.proquest.com/scholarly-journals/rasburicase-prevention-treatment-tumour-lysis/docview/1034901278/se-2?accountid=28018.
39. Niforatos JD, Zheutlin AR, Chaitoff A, et al. Things we do for no reason™: rasburicase for adult patients with tumor lysis syndrome. J Hosp Med 2021;16(7):424–7. Available at: https://onlinelibrary.wiley.com/doi/abs/10.12788/jhm.3618.
40. Ueng S. Rasburicase (elitek): a novel agent for tumor lysis syndrome. Proc Baylor Univ Med Cent 2005;18(3):275–9. Available at: https://www.tandfonline.com/doi/abs/10.1080/08998280.2005.11928082.
41. Abu-Alfa AK, Younes A. Tumor lysis syndrome and acute kidney injury: evaluation, prevention, and management. Am J Kidney Dis 2010;55(5):A4. Available at: https://www.clinicalkey.es/playcontent/1-s2.0-S0272638610006074.
42. Stewart AF,MD. Hypercalcemia associated with cancer. N Engl J Med 2005; 352(4):373–9. Available at: https://ezproxy.libraries.udmercy.edu/login?url=https://www.proquest.com/scholarly-journals/hypercalcemia-associated-with-cancer/docview/223933997/se-2?accountid=28018.
43. Walker J. Diagnosis and management of patients with hypercalcaemia. Nurs Older People 2015;27(4):22. Available at: https://ezproxy.libraries.udmercy.edu/

login?url=https://www.proquest.com/scholarly-journals/diagnosis-management-patients-with-hypercalcaemia/docview/1785295597/se-2?accountid=28018.

44. Gabriel J. Acute oncological emergencies. Nurs Stand 2012;27(4):35–41. Available at: https://www.ncbi.nlm.nih.gov/pubmed/23101297.

45. Rose M. Oncology in primary care. Philadelphia: Wolters Kluwer; 2013. Available at: https://ebookcentral.proquest.com/lib/[SITE_ID]/detail.action?docID=2031688.

46. Rosner MH, Dalkin AC. Onco-nephrology: the pathophysiology and treatment of malignancy-associated hypercalcemia. Clin J Am Soc Nephrol 2012;7(10): 1722–9. Available at: http://cjasn.asnjournals.org/content/7/10/1722.abstract.

47. Maier JD, Levine SN. Hypercalcemia in the intensive care unit. J Intensive Care Med 2015;30(5):235–52.

48. Lewis MA, Hendrickson AW, Moynihan TJ. Oncologic emergencies: pathophysiology, presentation, diagnosis, and treatment. CA: a Cancer J Clinicians 2011; 61(5):287–314. Available at: https://onlinelibrary.wiley.com/doi/abs/10.3322/caac.20124.

49. Jafari A, Rezaei-Tavirani M, Salimi M, et al. Oncological emergencies from pathophysiology and diagnosis to treatment: a narrative review. Social work Public Health 2020;35(8):689–709. Available at: https://www.tandfonline.com/doi/abs/10.1080/19371918.2020.1824844.

50. Halfdanarson TR, Hogan WJ, Moynihan TJ. Oncologic emergencies: diagnosis and treatment. Mayo Clin Proc 2006;81(6):835–48. https://doi.org/10.4065/81.6.835. Available at:.

51. Saunders Y, Ross JR, Broadley KE, et al. Systematic review of bisphosphonates for hypercalcaemia of malignancy. Palliat Med 2004;18(5):418–31. Available at: https://ezproxy.libraries.udmercy.edu/login?url=https://www.proquest.com/scholarly-journals/systematic-review-bisphosphonates-hypercalcaemia/docview/217818532/se-2?accountid=28018.

52. Minisola S, Pepe J, Piemonte S, et al. The diagnosis and management of hypercalcaemia. Br Med J (Online) 2015;350. n/a.Available at: https://ezproxy.libraries.udmercy.edu/login?url=https://www.proquest.com/scholarly-journals/diagnosis-management-hypercalcaemia/docview/1777763123/se-2?accountid=28018.

53. Sharma A, Einstein AJ, Vallakati A, et al. Risk of atrial fibrillation with use of oral and intravenous bisphosphonates. Am J Cardiol 2014;113(11):1815–21. https://doi.org/10.1016/j.amjcard.2014.03.008. Available at: https://ezproxy.libraries.udmercy.edu/login?url=https://www.proquest.com/scholarly-journals/risk-atrial-fibrillation-with-use-oral/docview/1524242034/se-2?accountid=28018.

54. Thandra K, Salah Z, Chawla S. Oncologic Emergencies—the old, the new, and the deadly. J Intensive Care Med 2020;35(1):3–13.

55. Hull CS, O'Rourke ME. Oncology-critical care nursing collaboration: recommendations for optimizing continuity of care of critically ill patients with cancer. Clin J Oncol Nurs 2007;11(6):925–7. Available at: https://ezproxy.libraries.udmercy.edu/login?url=https://www.proquest.com/scholarly-journals/oncology-critical-care-nursing-collaboration/docview/222742294/se-2?accountid=28018.

56. Maloney K, Denno M. Tumor lysis syndrome: prevention and detection to enhance patient safety. Clin J Oncol Nurs 2011;15(6):601–3. Available at: https://www.ncbi.nlm.nih.gov/pubmed/22119971.

57. Brigle K, Pierre A, Finley-Oliver E, et al. Myelosuppression, bone disease, and acute renal failure: evidence-based recommendations for oncologic emergencies. Clin J Oncol Nurs 2017;21(5 Suppl):60–76. Available at: https://www.ncbi.nlm.nih.gov/pubmed/28945730.

Palliative Care for Nephrology Patients in the Intensive Care Unit

Vivian Hemmat, MSN, AGACNP-BC, ACHPN,
Christine Corbett, DNP, APRN, FNP-BC, CNN-NP, FNKF*

KEYWORDS

- Palliative care • Kidney failure • Advance care planning • Goals of care
- Palliative nephrology • Supportive care • Conservative care • Acute kidney injury

KEY POINTS

- Nephrology and palliative care specialists are often consulted for patients with acute kidney failure in the ICU.
- Palliative care is supportive care for people with life-limiting illness and should be available for patients with kidney failure.
- Patients and families request prognostic information before starting dialysis.
- Shared decision making, goals of care discussions, and advance care planning ensure the treatment plan is in line with patient preferences through disease trajectory.
- Palliative care offers patient and family interdisciplinary support and symptom management to improve quality of life.

BACKGROUND

According to the National Kidney Foundation 2020 data, chronic kidney disease (CKD) affects more than 37 million Americans, with millions unaware of the diagnosis. Of those, more than 700,000 people progress to kidney failure.[1,2] The processes to determine persons appropriate for receiving dialysis have dramatically changed over the past 60 plus years. Historically, middle-aged healthy males (no diagnosis of hypertension) were selected for dialysis consideration by committee due to limited resources and high costs of treatment.[3–5]

Today, dialysis is offered to much older adults including those with multiple comorbid conditions, including heart failure, dementia, and cancer inside and outside the hospital setting.[6,7] Despite an Institute of Medicine report in 1990 indicating patient reports of poor quality of life (QOL) with dialysis, and recommendations for nephrologists

University Health Truman Medical Center, 2301 Holmes Street, Kansas City, MO 64108, USA
* Corresponding author.
E-mail address: Christine.corbett@uhkc.org

Crit Care Nurs Clin N Am 34 (2022) 467–479
https://doi.org/10.1016/j.cnc.2022.07.003
0899-5885/22/© 2022 Elsevier Inc. All rights reserved.

to be selective with dialysis suggestions, dialysis continues to remain the default treatment option for kidney failure in the United States, leaving patients with great symptom burden and poor QOL.[7]

QOL and symptom assessments of patients with CKD reveal that many patients suffer greatly from symptom burden related to kidney disease, often more so than patients diagnosed with cancer receiving therapy.[8–14] The United States Renal Data System (USRDS)[15] revealed that morbidity and mortality rates are high and continue to increase in patients diagnosed with CKD and/or kidney failure, with tripled mortality rates in those older than 85 years. The USRDS also shows that patients are withdrawing from dialysis at higher rates, but unfortunately, receiving end-of-life care hospitalized (2016).

In addition, the in-hospital mortality rates of patients admitted to the ICU receiving renal replacement therapies (RRTs) (dialysis and continuous renal replacement therapy) are more than 60% according to Uchino and colleagues (2005).[16] Another study surveying patients who survived their ICU admission found an out-of-hospital mortality rate of 52.6%, and of those survivors, nearly 30% rated a very poor QOL.[17] These studies indicate additional need for shared decision making, prognostication, and palliative care support.

DISCUSSION

Palliative care is a unique medical specialty that emphasizes care of the total person, physical, emotional, social, and spiritual. Teams are typically interdisciplinary and may include physicians, advanced practice nurses, registered nurses, social workers, chaplains, pharmacists, and other specialists with a goal to prevent and relieve suffering and to support the best QOL for patient and family regardless of the stage of disease or treatment choices. An inpatient palliative care team helps manage symptoms and spends time with the patient and family to establish goals of care and discuss advance care planning. The team sees patients and families over repeated hospitalizations, works to build trust and rapport over time, understands the history and progression of patient's disease, and reviews previous goals-of-care discussions to help address current needs/wishes (Center to Advance Palliative Care [CAPC], Campbell, Nelson, Weissman, Fast Facts and Concepts #253, n.d.) (**Box 1**).

Box 1
Reasons to consider palliative care for persons with kidney disease per CAPC (2020)[18]; RPA (2010)[19]; and Pathways Project (2020)[20] include

ICU admission and life-threatening condition

Difficult symptom control

Declining function

Multiple hospitalizations

Uncertainty of prognosis/goals of care

Advance care planning

Family distress impairing surrogate decision making

Decision about life-sustaining technology/dialysis discussion

Previous palliative care referral

Prognosis and the ability to communicate prognosis to persons with kidney disease is imperative for informed decision making, whether patients are diagnosed with acute kidney injury or end-stage kidney disease. Unfortunately, the literature reports that patients are often not aware of disease severity or are given a false sense of hope with dialysis discussion and suggestion.[6,9,21–23] Use of prognostic indicators to determine patient suitability for dialysis are also underutilized, again allowing for a sense of false hope for patients when they are considering options. Data show that 22.5% of Medicare patients who start dialysis die within 30 days, 44.2% within 6 months, and 54.5% within a year.[22] The Center to Advance Palliative Care (CAPC) offers guidance for nurses and providers wishing to expand their communication skills when holding difficult conversations with patients and families.[24,25]

Guidelines, including *The Shared Decision Making in the Appropriate Initiation of and Withdrawal from Dialysis,* have existed for over two decades providing useful recommendations for nurses and providers in holding goals-of-care conversations through shared decision making.[19] The guideline outlines persons who may have poor prognosis on hemodialysis, discusses the importance of holding conversations with patients, and facilitates advance care planning[19] (**Box 2**).

A study by Zhou and colleagues (2012)[26] found the patients with the highest intensive care unit (ICU) mortality included those with severe AKI, increased baseline creatinine, sepsis, ventilation, severe pancreatitis, three or more failed organ systems, and ICU length of stay. Information such as this should be used when holding discussions regarding prognosis with patients, if able, and friends/families.

It is important to discuss a potentially poor survival rate or QOL when proceeding with hemodialysis, for patients who fit the above listed criteria. The Coalition of Supportive Care of Kidney Patients[20] designed a prognostic aid for providers and nurses to determine patient prognosis based on certain indicators (with permission and in the public domain). Note that this information is provided to guide discussions for patients with advanced CKD; however, it may also translate to the ICU setting, especially when those patients present with the indicators on **Fig. 1**.

Other prognostic indicators (**Fig. 2**) include the Charlson Comorbidity Index, Karnofsky Performance Status Scale, the Surprise Question, and the diagnosis of serious illness.

The Charlson Comorbidity Index

The Charlson Comorbidity Index (https://www.mdcalc.com/charlson-comorbidity-index-cci) is a useful tool that uses comorbidities in determining 10-year survival

---

Box 2
Guidelines from *The Shared Decision Making in the Appropriate Initiation of and Withdrawal from Dialysis*

Establishing a shared decision-making relationship

Informing patients of prognosis/options

Facilitating advance care planning

Making a decision to not initiate or to discontinue dialysis

Resolving conflicts about what dialysis decisions to make

Providing effective palliative care

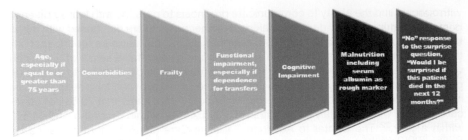

Fig. 1. Indicators of patients that may translate to ICU setting.

rate.[27] The nurse or provider can use the calculator to input patient comorbidities and age to receive the 10-year life expectancy.

The Karnofsky Performance Status uses functional status, including independence or reliance on support with activities of daily living.[28] The lower the Karnofsky score, the poorer the prognosis and survival rate. The tool is used by palliative care clinicians and nephrologists and is supported through the[19] *Shared Decision-Making* guidelines.[19] The Guideline suggests *patients with a Karnofsky of less than 40 are not good dialysis candidates* (2010). This is important for patients diagnosed with CKD, or AKI and treatment options, including dialysis.

Surprise Question: Utilizing the guideline's "surprise" question, *Will I be surprised if this patient died in the next 12 months?* assists nurses and providers in predicting disease trajectory and dialysis discussion and/or palliative care referral.[19,29] The surprise question can guide treatment even in the acute setting.

Serious Illness is defined as "a health condition that carries a high risk of mortality AND either negatively impacts a person's daily life function or quality of life, OR excessively strains their caregivers"[30(pS-8)]. Diagnoses included within this definition are kidney failure, dementia, chronic obstructive pulmonary disease, congestive heart failure, peripheral arterial disease, malignant cancer, or leukemia.[30] Several palliative nephrologists suggest a consult for palliative and supportive care for all patients diagnosed

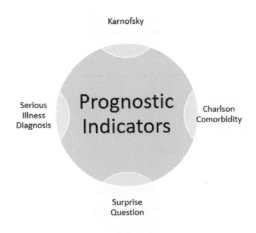

Fig. 2. Other prognostic indicators.

with serious illness.[20,29,31,32] The Kidney Disease: Improving Global Outcomes suggests serious illness identification to trigger a goals-of-care conversation. Once patient wishes and values are determined, symptom support should be offered.[33]

Symptom Burden with Chronic Kidney Disease/Kidney Failure

The following are common symptoms associated with kidney failure (**Box 3**), which lend the need for additional support, such as palliative care, for improved QOL.[34,35] Germain and colleagues[6] determined many elderly patients, if given the choice, would prefer improved QOL over life extension (2018).

Unfortunately, many patients diagnosed with kidney disease were not informed of the degree of symptom burden they may experience on hemodialysis or of their prognosis.[36] In addition, some patients expressed the inability to make an informed decision to start dialysis. According to the same study by Saeed and colleagues[36] of 397 patients undergoing dialysis, the patients who were best informed did not regret the decision to start hemodialysis. There were 21% who had regrets and were not given information regarding symptom burden or who felt pressured by family to start dialysis[36]; this should be a consideration in the ICU setting given the number of patients who start dialysis during an acute event and do not recover kidney function after discharge.

The USRDS study (2021)[37] (n = 1000 patients on hemodialysis) found the most common self-reported symptoms and frequency shown in **Fig. 3**.

In addition to symptom burden and poor QOL for some patients who choose hemodialysis, frequent hospitalizations may be required to manage vascular access, cardiac complications, or symptoms.[15,38]

The following are the symptom assessment tools useful for persons with CKD or kidney failure. The Edmonton Symptom Assessment Revised-*Renal* is an 11 symptom Likert scale that includes pain, gastrointestinal issues, and depression. The Beck Depression Inventory and the Patient Health Questionnaire are great tools to assess anxiety and depression, which occur frequently in patients with kidney disease. Assessing for symptom burden and addressing appropriately through pharmacologic and nonpharmacologic methods can improve QOL.

Pharmacologic Management of Symptoms for Patients with Chronic Kidney Disease/Kidney Failure

In 2019, Sara Davidson, MD, a palliative nephrologist from Alberta, Canada, released an article entitled, "Recommendations for the Care of Patients Receiving Conservative Kidney Management." This publication serves as a guide for the management of

---

Box 3
Common symptoms associated with kidney failure

Pain

Pruritis

Depression

Gastrointestinal symptoms

Insomnia

Fatigue

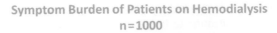

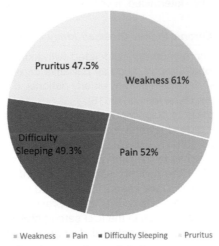

Fig. 3. Symptom burden of patients on hemodialysis.

persons who choose to forego dialysis or other aggressive therapies for kidney failure. Included are symptom management recommendations.

Pain medications for use in CKD and end-stage renal disease are listed in (**Fig. 4**); this was developed by the Center for the Coalition of Supportive Care of Kidney Patients.[20]

Shared decision making should be the cornerstone before dialysis initiation especially in the critical care setting. In addition, shared decision making should guide elevated support through referral to palliative care specialists, for patients with multiple comorbid conditions and serious illness, and for RRT decision making and symptom management.[19,29,31,36,39–43]

Palliative care professionals seek to match patient preferences with treatment plans through goals-of-care discussions. Goals-of-care discussions typically take place when there is a change in health status and the treatment pathway needs to be determined or re-evaluated; this may be with a new diagnosis of a life-limiting illness, with progression of disease or decline in health status, as patient approaches end of life, or if there is a change in patient preferences. Discussions may be with patient and/or family depending on patient's wishes and capacity and may include palliative care team members, the primary team, and other specialty medical teams involved in patient's care. Before a goals-of-care discussion, providers should review data including relevant medical history, current treatments and any positive or negative effects, treatment options being proposed, and prognosis with and without continued disease-directed treatments and determine medical opinions about the utility of proposed or current treatments among consultants and the primary team. A palliative care team will also seek out patient/family psychosocial data that may impact decision making as well as what has transpired in any prior meetings.[44]

The next step in a goals-of-care discussion is to determine patient/family's understanding and perspective regarding their health status. Then the provider can offer new information or correct misunderstandings and answer questions. The provider leading the discussion should offer a succinct summary of the current condition

Pain Medications in CKD/ESRD

Recommended	Use with Caution	Do Not Use
Acetaminophen	**Tramadol** Limit dose to 50 mg BID. Higher doses have been used but caution needs to be taken since pharmacokinetics are not well established.	**Morphine**
Hydromorphone Hydromorphone is potentially unsafe if the patient stops dialysis OR is CKD stage 4 or 5. The kidney-excreted active metabolite, hydromorphone-3-glucuronide, build ups because it is not adequately cleared in worsening CKD.	**Hydrocodone/Oxycodone** Insufficient pharmacokinetic evidence to establish safety in CKD, but literature reports use without major adverse effects.	**Codeine**
Fentanyl	**Desipramine/Nortriptyline** Alternative to treat neuropathic pain, but more adverse effects than gabapentin and pregabalin.	**Meperidine**
Methadone		**Propoxyphene** Renally excreted metabolites accumulate in CKD causing neurotoxicity.
Gabapentin Doses in ESRD up to 300mg/d are generally considered safe, but higher doses should be used with caution; note that gabapentin use for neuropathic pain is off-label but effectiveness has been documented.		
Pregabalin Doses up to 100 mg/d are generally considered safe in ESRD.		

Fig. 4. Pain medications in CKD and end-stage renal disease (ESRD).

without using medical jargon and taking into account patient's health literacy and cultural/religious considerations. Focus should be on issues of most importance, usually function/quality/time: "Give a 'bottom-line' statement: 'getting worse,' 'not going to improve, 'dying and time is likely very short'"; "Once the goal(s) is/are established, you can then review the patient's current treatments…" Anything that will not help meet the goals should be discussed for potential discontinuation.[45,46]

Another important aspect of palliative care is *advance care planning*. Advance care planning encourages patients to complete a Durable Power of Attorney for health care (DPOA) and document preferences related to the types of medical interventions desired in the future in an advance directive (AD). A DPOA for health care designates a persons to make medical decisions for a patient *only* when the patient is deemed incapacitated. Only a capacitated patient can name a DPOA/complete documentation, and patients should be encouraged to name someone who will honor the patient's preferences. Patients should also be encouraged to share their preferences with the DPOA and to let them know they have been selected to perform this duty. A health care provider or a social worker can assist with completion of a DPOA document. Refer to hospital policies and state laws related to scope of practice regarding determining capacity.

The purpose of an AD is to discover and list medical interventions a patient would or would not wish to have in the future, such as resuscitation in the event of cardiac or respiratory arrest or prolonged life support. Through goals-of-care discussions, it is helpful to discuss a person's understanding and desires of QOL, list those medical interventions desired, under what circumstances, and for how long. The AD may be updated based on patient preferences or change in health status.[20,47–49] The Center for Practical Bioethics (2020)[47] offers the "Caring Conversations" workbook free of charge (https://www.practicalbioethics.org/resources/caring-conversations.html), and it is available in both English and Spanish.

TRANSITIONAL CARE

For those patients, or families honoring patient wishes in the ICU, who choose not to proceed with dialysis or other aggressive measures, or who are found to be poor candidates for dialysis, supportive, conservative kidney management (CKM) may provide the best benefit. For patients uncertain about dialysis, dialysis should be offered as a time-limited trial, with the expectation of planning the duration and expected follow-up (ie, 30, 60, or 90 days). The *Shared Decision-Making* guidelines suggest "… a time-limited trial of dialysis for patients requiring dialysis, but who have an uncertain prognosis, or for whom a consensus cannot be reached about providing dialysis."[19(p4)] Patients should also be offered a central venous catheter as access during the trial. If the patient chooses to continue dialysis, plans for permanent access can be made. In addition, for those patients who choose not to proceed with dialysis after the trial, transitional care to hospice should be suggested.[20,32]

CKM, supportive care, and active medical management without dialysis is a holistic, person-centered approach to kidney failure without dialysis or transplant. Although there are few outpatient programs across the nation to support patients who forego dialysis, there are resources and international programs to model, including Alberta, Canada's Conservative Kidney Management,[50] Kidney Health Australia,[51] and the US' Pathways Project.[20] Moss and colleagues[32] edited the text, *Palliative Care in Nephrology*, which went to press in 2020 and is a useful blend of palliative care and nephrology in decision making.

Hospice is end-of-life care that provides symptom management and support for patients and families and is available in a variety of settings, including in some hospitals.

Eligibility requirements vary based on disease-specific criteria and/or overall prognosis, but generally a prognosis of 6 months or less qualifies an individual for hospice services.[18]

Comfort care is end-of-life care provided within the hospital setting for patients actively dying and for whom transfer home with family, to a hospice house, or to a long-term care facility may result in death in transit. ICU nurses are often the caregivers for dying patients and should recommend a palliative care team referral to assist with symptom management and patient and family support.

DEFINITIONS

Palliative care: Palliative care is specialized medical care for people living with a serious illness. This type of care is focused on providing relief from the symptoms and stress of the illness. The goal is to improve QOL for both the patient and the family. Palliative care teams work collaboratively with other medical professionals to provide an extra layer of support. Such care is appropriate at any age and at any stage in a serious illness, and it can be provided along with curative treatment.[18]

Conservative kidney management: CKM, conservative care, kidney supportive care, and active medical management without dialysis are interchangeable terms to describe a type of care for persons with advanced kidney disease who choose to forego dialysis or transplantation but seek treatment of numerous debilitating symptoms and continued CKD management.[32]

Hospice: "Hospice care is a philosophy of supportive and palliative care provided to people at the end of their life. The focus of hospice care is on the management of symptoms, providing comfort care and supporting quality of life rather than curative treatments."[52]

Capacity: "Patients have medical decision-making capacity if they can demonstrate understanding of the situation, appreciation of the consequences of their decision, and reasoning in their thought process, and if they can communicate their wishes."[53]

Advance directive: An AD documents patient wishes and goals of care for the future. AD includes the opportunity to name a DPOA and specific preferences related to medical interventions a patient would or would not want in the future (Center for Practical Bioethics).

DPOA: DPOA documents persons chosen by the patient to act on behalf of the patient should the patient not be able to make decisions on their own (ie, intubated, sedated, lacking capacity to make decisions[54][p46]).

Out of Hospital Do Not Resuscitate: A document that indicates a patient's request not to be resuscitated in the event of cardiac/respiratory arrest when that person is in a nonhospital setting.

Physician Orders for Life Sustaining Treatment, Medical Orders for Life Sustaining Treatment, Transportable Physician Orders for Patient Preferences: A document that translates the values expressed in an AD into immediately active medical orders. This document aims to provide continuity of care for patients across all care settings (eg, hospitals, hospice, long-term care, and home) and transfers with the patient throughout the health care system. Title of document varies with different regions.[55]

SUMMARY

A collaborative relationship between critical care nursing and the inpatient palliative care team provides a patient-centered approach to care for individuals with kidney failure. Critical care nurses may be the first to identify patients appropriate for palliative care referral and encourage the primary team to place a consult based upon criteria listed in this article. These nurses may be most aware of those patients who return repeatedly to the hospital, have distressing symptoms or a decline in function over time, and would benefit from a goals of care discussion. Critical care nurses may have valuable information related to patient preferences shared with the bedside nurse but not discussed with the primary team, nephrology, or family. Because palliative care offers continuity as a patient moves throughout the hospital or returns to the hospital, ICU nurses can assist in encouraging early palliative care team consults to maintain that continuity.

CLINICS CARE POINTS

- Patients with kidney failure request prognostic information and dialysis survival rates before initiating treatment. ICU nurses can help identify need and encourage discussion between patient, family, and provider.

- Patients diagnosed with end-stage kidney failure or acute kidney injury in the ICU benefit from a palliative care referral for symptom management, goals of care discussions, and advance care planning. Critical care nurses can help identify those patients who would benefit from a palliative care referral and encourage providers to consult the palliative care team.

- Critical care nurses are often the caregivers for dying patients. Nurses should encourage a palliative care team referral to assist with referral for hospice care, end-of-life symptom management, and family support.

DISCLOSURE

C. Corbett has participated in a PCORI grant submission through George Washington University and the Coalition for Supportive Care of Kidney Patients.

REFERENCES

1. World Health Organization. Palliative care key facts. 2020. https://www.who.int/news-room/fact-sheets/detail/palliative-care. Accessed January 11, 2022.
2. NKF, 2020. Chronic kidney disease (CKD) - Symptoms, causes, treatment. https://www.kidney.org/atoz/content/about-chronic-kidney-disease. Accessed October 1, 2022.
3. Alexander S. They decide who lives, who dies. Life 1962;102–25.
4. Counts C, American Nephrology Nurses Association. Core curriculum for nephrology nursing. Counts. In: C.S., editor. Pitman. New Jersey: Anthony J. Jannetti, Inc; 2020.
5. Blagg CR. The early history of dialysis for chronic renal failure in the United States: a view from Seattle. Am J Kidney Dis 2007;49(3):482–96.
6. Germain MJ, Davison SN, Moss AH. When enough is enough: the nephrologist's responsibility in ordering dialysis treatments. Am J Kidney Dis 2018;58(1):135–43.
7. Wong S, McFarland LV, Liu CF, et al. Care practices for patients with advanced kidney disease who forgo maintenance dialysis. JAMA Intern Med 2019;179(3):305–13.
8. Davison SN. End-of-life care preferences and needs: perceptions of patients with chronic kidney disease. Clin J Am Soc Nephrol 2010;5:195–204.

9. Davison SN. The ethics of end-of-life care for patients with ESRD. Clin J Am Soc Nephrol 2012;7:2049–57.
10. Davison SN, Jhangri GS, Holley JL, et al. Nephrologists' reported preparedness for end-of-life decision-making. Clin J Am Soc Nephrol 2006;1(6):1256–62.
11. Grubbs V, Moss AH, Cohen LM, et al. A palliative approach to dialysis care: a patient-centered transition to the end-of-life. Clin J Am Soc Nephrol 2014;9: 2203–9.
12. Moss AH. Palliative care in patients with kidney disease and cancer. In: Onconephrology curriculum. Washington DC: American Society of Nephrology; 2016. Available at: https://www.asn-online.org/education/distancelearning/curricula/onco/Chapter19.pdf.
13. National Kidney Foundation. More palliative care options needed for dialysis patients. 2014. https://www.kidney.org/news/newsroom/nr/More-Palliative-Care-Options-Needed. Accessed January 10, 2022.
14. Weisbord SD, Fried LF, Arnold RM, et al. Prevalence, severity and importance of physical and emotional symptoms in chronic hemodialysis patients. J Am Soc Nephrol 2005;16:2487–94.
15. U. S. Renal Data System. USRDS annual data report: atlas of chronic kidney disease and end-stage renal disease in the United States. Bethesda, MD: National Institutes of Health, National Institute of Diabetes and Digestive and Kidney Diseases; 2016. Available at: http://www.usrds.org/adr.aspx.
16. Uchino S, Kellum JA, Bellomo R, et al. Acute renal failure in critically ill patients; A multinational, multicenter study. J Am Med Assoc 2005;294(7):813–8.
17. Johansen KL, Smith MW, Unruh ML, et al. Predictors of health utility among 60-day survivors of acute kidney injury in the veterans affairs/national institutes of health acute renal failure trial network study. Clin J Am Soc Nephrol 2010;5(8): 1366–72.
18. Centers to Advance Palliative Care. CAPC palliative care referral criteria. 2020. Available at: https://www.capc.org/toolkits/patient-identification-and-assessment/. Accessed March 18, 2022.
19. Renal Physicians Association. Shared decision-making in the appropriate initiation of and withdrawal from dialysis-clinical practice guideline. 2nd edition. Rockville (MD): Renal Physicians Association; 2010. Available at: https://cdn.ymaws.com/www.renalmd.org/resource/resmgr/Store/Shared_Decision_Making_Recom.pdf.
20. Pathways Project. Change Package - Just Right Care. 2020. https://gwu.app.box.com/s/d9jqjhk7fxf0bqidlqu21lhlzmy97sdw. Accessed February 1, 2022.
21. Verberne WR, Geers T, Jellema WT, et al. Comparative survival among older adults with advanced kidney disease managed conservatively versus with dialysis. Clin J Am Soc Nephrol 2016;11. https://doi.org/10.2215/CJN.07510715.
22. Wachterman MW, O'Hare AM, Rahman O, et al. One-year mortality after dialysis initiation among older adults. J Am Med Assoc Intern Med 2019;179(7):987–90.
23. Saaed F, Epstein RM, Monk RD, et al. Dialysis regret: Prevalence and correlates. Clinical Journal of the American Society of Nephrology 2020;15(7):957–63.
24. Centers to Advance Palliative Care. Communication skills for conversations about serious illness. 2020. https://www.capc.org. Accessed August 1, 2022.
25. Centers to Advance Palliative Care. The case for palliative care. 2020. https://www.capc.org/the-case-for-palliative-care/. Accessed August 1, 2022.
26. Zhou J, Yang L, Zhang K, et al. Risk factors for the prognosis of acute kidney injury under the Acute Kidney Injury Network definition: a retrospective, multicenter study. Nephrology 2012;17(4):330–7.

27. MD plus Calculator. Charleson comorbidity Index. 2020. Available at: https://www.mdcalc.com/charlson-comorbidity-index-cci.
28. National Palliative Care Research Center. Karnofski performance scale Index. 2013. http://www.npcrc.org/files/news/karnofsky_performance_scale.pdf. Accessed September 1, 2022.
29. O'Hare AM, Song MK, Tamura MK, et al. Research priorities for palliative care for older adults with advanced Chronic Kidney Disease. J Palliat Med 2018;20(5):453–60.
30. Kelley AS, Bollens-Lund E. Identifying the population with serious illness: the "denominator" challenge. J Palliat Med 2018;21(2):S7–16. https://doi.org/10.1089/jpm.2017.0548.
31. Grubbs V. Palliative dialysis. In: Moss AH, Lupu DE, Armistead NC, et al, editors. Palliative care in nephrology. New York, NY: Oxford University Press; 2020. p. 220–6.
32. Moss AH, Lupu D, Armistead N, et al. Palliative care in nephrology. New York, NY: Oxford University Press; 2020.
33. Davison SN, Levin A, Moss AH, et al. Kidney disease: improving global outcomes. Executive summary of the KDIGO controversies conference on supportive care in chronic kidney disease: developing a roadmap to improving quality care. Kidney Int 2015;88(3):447–59.
34. American Nephrology Nurses Association. Position statement: nephrology nurse's role in palliative and end-of-life care. 2018. http://anna.inurse.com/download/reference/health/position/palliativeCare.pdf. Accessed November 1, 2022.
35. Han Y, Rajesh B, Hirth RA, et al. Assessment of prescription analgesic use in older adults with and without chronic kidney disease and outcomes. J Am Med Assoc 2020;3(9). https://doi.org/10.1001/jamanetworkopen.2020.16839.
36. Saaed F, Epstein RM, Monk RD, et al. Dialysis regret: prevalence and correlates. Clin J Am Soc Nephrol 2020;15(7):957–63.
37. U. S. Renal Data System. Patient experience: end of life care for patients with ESRD. 2021. https://adr.usrds.org/2020/end-stage-renal-disease/12-patient-experience-end-of-life-care-for-patients-with-esrd. Accessed November 1, 2022.
38. National Kidney Foundation, More palliative care options needed for dialysis patients. 2014. Available at: https://www.kidney.org/news/newsroom/nr/More-Palliative-Care-Options-Needed.
39. Brown MA, Collett GK, Josland EA, et al. CKD in elderly patients managed without dialysis: survival, symptoms, and quality of life. Clin J Am Soc Nephrol 2015;10(2):260–8.
40. Cohen LM, Ruthhazer R, Moss AH, et al. Predicting six-month mortality for patients who are on maintenance hemodialysis. Clin J Am Soc Nephrol 2010;5(1):72–9.
41. Russell JS, Lupu D, Seliger S, et al. Providing supportive care to patients with kidney disease. Nephrology News & Issues. 2016. http://www.nephrologynews.com/providing-supportive-care-to-patients-with-kidney-disease/. Accessed August 1, 2022.
42. Schueller K, Lupu DE. Unmet palliative care needs of patients with kidney disease and consequences. In: Moss AH, Lupu DE, Armistead NC, et al, editors. Palliative care in nephrology. New York, NY: Oxford University Press; 2020. p. 21–35.
43. Smith V, Potts C, Wellard S, et al. Integrating renal and palliative care project: a nurse-led initiative. Ren Soc Australasia J 2015;11:35–40.

44. Arnold Robert M. Quill, tim, and weissman, david. Fast facts and Concepts #222. Preparing for the family meeting. Available at: https://www.mypcnow.org. Accessed March 18, 2022.

45. Arnold Robert M. Quill, tim, and weissman, david. Fast facts and Concepts #223. The family meeting: starting the conversation. Available at: https://www.mypcnow.org. Accessed March 18, 2022.

46. Arnold Robert M. Quill, Tim, and Weissman, David. Fast Facts and Concepts #227. The family meeting: end of life goal setting and future planning. Available at: https://www.mypcnow.org. Accessed March 18, 2022.

47. Center for Practical Bioethics. Caring conversations. 2020. https://practicalbioethics.org/programs/advance-care-planning.html. Accessed August 1, 2022.

48. Coalition for Supportive Care of Kidney Patients. For professionals. 2020. https://www.kidneysupportivecare.org/. Accessed October 1, 2022.

49. Davison SN. Fast Facts and Concepts #162. Advance care planning in chronic illness. Available at: https://www.mypcnow.org. Accessed March 18, 2022.

50. CKM, 2020. Conservative Kidney Management. Available at: https://www.ckmcare.com/. Accessed December 1, 2022.

51. Kidney Health Australia, 2020. Comprehensive Conservative Care. Available at: https://kidney.org.au/your-kidneys/treatment/comprehensive-conservative-care Accessed January 12, 2022

52. Ferrell BR, Coyle N, Paice JA. *Oxford Textbook of Palliative Nursing*. 4th Ed. NY: Oxford University Press; 2015.

53. Barstow C, Shahan B, Roberts M. Evaluating Medical Decision-Making Capacity in Practice. American Family Physician 2018;98(1):40–6.

54. Wiegand DL, Russo MM. Ethical Considerations. In: Dahlin, Lynch, editors. *Core Curriculum for the Advanced Practice Hospice and Palliative Registered Nurse*. Hospice and Palliative Nurses Association; 2013. p. 39–59.

55. Citko J, Moss A, Carley M, et al. Fast Facts and Concepts #178. The national polst paradigm initiative. Available at: https://www.mypcnow.org. Accessed March 18, 2022.

Kidney Disease and Sars-coV-2 Infection
Challenges and Considerations for Nursing

Sherry Rivera, DNP, APRN, ANP-C, FNKF*, Clair Millet, DNP, APRN, PHCNS-BC

KEYWORDS

- Kidney disease • COVID-19 infection • Treatment challenges
- Infection control measures • Acute kidney injury • Kidney transplant
- Sars-coV-2 infection

KEY POINTS

- The COVID-19 pandemic has significantly affected the morbidity and mortality of patients with kidney disease worldwide.
- The challenges encountered during the COVID-19 pandemic have presented valuable lessons learned for future pandemics, other public health emergencies, and disasters.
- The COVID-19 pandemic has further exposed the need for more nurses to be knowledgeable about the care of kidney disease.
- Nursing leaders are needed to identify innovative methods for educating the nursing workforce that is specialized in nephrology care.

INTRODUCTION

The novel Coronavirus Disease (COVID-19) was declared a pandemic by the World Health Organization on March 11, 2020. A national emergency was declared in the United States concerning the COVID-19 outbreak on March 13, 2020. The COVID-19 pandemic has significantly affected the morbidity and mortality of patients with kidney disease across the spectrum of disease worldwide. Sars-coV-2 infection has been linked to the development of acute kidney injury (AKI) and worsening of underlying kidney function. The long-term sequelae of sars-coV-2 infection and kidney disease remain to be seen. Before the COVID-19 pandemic, approximately 15% of the population in the United States had kidney disease with 1 in 3 adults at risk for developing the disease.[1] According to the National Kidney Foundation (2021), approximately 90% of individuals with kidney disease are unaware of their disease status. A lack of

Louisiana State University Health New Orleans School of Nursing, Nurse Practitioner Program, 1900 Gravier Street, New Orleans, LA 70112, USA
* Corresponding author.
E-mail address: srive4@lsuhsc.edu

Crit Care Nurs Clin N Am 34 (2022) 481–490
https://doi.org/10.1016/j.cnc.2022.07.007

awareness leads to poor health outcomes due to missed opportunities for treatment and preventative efforts. There is concern that there will be an increase in the number of individuals affected with kidney disease because of the long-term effects of sars-coV-2 infection.

The COVID-19 pandemic presented many challenges for nurses in the hospital and outpatient settings. Nurses in the hospital setting provided care to many individuals with kidney disease and sars-coV-2 infection. According to the United States Renal Data System (2021), out of 302,128 Medicare recipients with end-stage renal disease (ESRD) receiving dialysis treatments, 47,860 individuals were diagnosed with COVID-19 by the end of December 2020. The cumulative incidence of COVID-19 diagnosis during that same period was 15.8% with 14% in white individuals, 16.6% in black individuals, and 18.7% in individuals of other races/ethnicities.[2] Almost 8% of Medicare recipients with chronic kidney disease (CKD) were diagnosed with COVID-19 by the end of 2020.[3] More than 9% of Medicare recipients with a kidney transplant were diagnosed with COVID-19 by the end of December 2020.[2] Among outpatient dialysis clinics more than 20% of patients had contracted sars-coV-2 infection by the end of 2020.[2] Overall, the rates of hospitalization for Medicare recipients with CKD were 3 times higher than recipients without CKD.[2] At the highest, the hospitalization rates for individuals with ESRD receiving dialysis ranged from 4 to 6 admissions per 1000.[3] The hospitalization rate among individuals with kidney transplant ranged from 0.6 to 3.2 admissions per 1000.[2] The significance of nursing's interaction with individuals with kidney disease should not be underestimated. Nurses provided care to individuals infected with the sars-coV-2 infection and kidney disease across multiple settings. Each nursing encounter with individual patients and their families is an opportunity to increase awareness of disease status and to assist preventative efforts to reduce the prevalence of kidney disease and improve the overall population health.

Nurses who are knowledgeable regarding the care of individuals with kidney disease are vitally important to improving health outcomes. As seen during the COVID-19 pandemic, nurses are extremely important for the delivery of quality health care. A shortage of more than 900,000 nurses is anticipated by the year 2030.[4] Nephrology nurses require specialized training, and the shortage of nephrology nurses trained to provide dialysis has been ongoing for more than a decade. The number of individuals receiving dialysis has been steadily rising for more than 20 years. Since 2009, there has been a 91% increase in the number of individuals that receive in-center hemodialysis.[2] Because the number of individuals receiving dialysis increases, the need for nurses trained in dialysis also increases. The nursing shortage has been affecting nephrology nursing for many years. Since 2004, 5% to 7% of outpatient dialysis nursing positions have remained unfilled and does not account for variability in location, and inpatient or transplant clinic positions that are available.[4] Nephrology nursing shortages have had a significant impact on the delivery of care to individuals with requiring dialysis treatments due to the sars-coV-2 infection. During the initial stages of the pandemic, the need for dialysis treatments in the hospital for individuals acutely ill with sars-coV-2 infection rapidly overwhelmed available resources including dialysis nurses, machines, and supplies for acute dialysis treatments and continuous renal replacement therapy (CRRT). Boyle and colleagues (2022) reported the number of bedside hemodialysis treatments tripled and patient days for continuous renal replacement (CRRT) doubled. Nurses and other clinic staff were at a heightened risk for contracting infection due to recurrent and prolonged exposure that led to staffing shortages due to illness.[5,6] The ongoing shortage of trained dialysis nurses, the significant increase in the number of dialysis nurses needed to deliver the overwhelming number of acute dialysis treatments and staff the outpatient dialysis clinics, and the significant number of dialysis nurses that contracted the sars-coV-2 infection created a scheduling nightmare that ultimately pushed dialysis nurses to the limit, requiring superpower strength for survival. The COVID-19 pandemic has further exposed the extensive need for more nurses to be knowledgeable about infectious disease and the care of kidney disease. It was evident that nurses require specialized training to administer dialysis.

Background

The COVID-19 pandemic has been linked to the development of AKI, collapsing glomerulopathy, acute tubular necrosis (ATN), progression of CKD, and higher rates of infection among patients with ESRD and kidney transplant. In the United States, AKI occurred more frequently in patients with underlying CKD (57%) before sars-co-V-2 infection than those without a history of CKD (28%).[7] The incidence of AKI related to sars-coV-2 infection was variable and was reported from 20% to 57% of hospitalized patients depending on the study.[8–12] Higher rates of AKI have been noted in the United States when compared with other countries and have been attributed to higher rates of comorbid diseases such as diabetes mellitus, CKD, and hypertension in the United States.[8] However, the presence of comorbid diseases alone does not account for all cases of AKI. Moledina and colleagues[9] (2021) demonstrated that COVID-19 is highly associated with AKI even after adjustment for the presence of comorbid conditions, demographic data, current medications, and laboratory results (n = 2600 patients). Variable definitions of AKI have also been a contributing factor to the variability in reported incidence rates.[8] In a retrospective observational study conducted by Chan and colleagues (2021), out of almost 4000 hospitalized patients with sars-coV-2 infection, 46% developed AKI with 19% requiring dialysis and 35% of patients did not regain kidney function at the time of discharge. AKI is an independent risk factor for mortality in COVID-19 patients. Poorer health outcomes and increased rates of mortality have been linked to sars-coV-2 infection among patients with AKI and/or kidney disease.

The exact pathophysiology of kidney failure in COVID-19 is unclear. Multiple mechanisms can contribute to the development of AKI related to sars-coV-2 infection. Immune system overaction, complement activation, release of cytokines, angiotensin II overactivation, and other inflammatory markers can lead to organ dysfunction, hypotension, acute heart failure, and cardiomyopathy due to cardiorenal syndrome. The development of a hypercoagulable state can also occur. Prerenal causes include azotemia related to intravascular volume depletion, and ATN due to hypotension, and shock. Sepsis can trigger multiple pathophysiologic mechanisms contributing to the development of AKI. The utilization of multiple commonly used medications such as antibiotics, nonsteroidal anti-inflammatory medications, antivirals, and others can cause acute interstitial nephritis. Endothelial dysfunction leads to the development of a hypercoagulable state, leading to ischemia and infarction within the kidneys, other organs, and the vasculature. Direct invasion of the kidney by the sars-coV-2 infection can lead to the development of several glomerulopathies.

Histologic findings of sars-coV-2 infection include ATN most commonly, glomerulosclerosis, myoglobin cast nephropathy, thrombotic microangiopathy, crescentic glomerulonephritis, and cortical necrosis.[8] Initial postmortem autopsy results identified diffuse proximal tubular necrosis from ischemia or the presence of sars-coV-2 infection of the epithelial cells in the kidney.[13] The study conducted by Hessler and colleagues (2021) evaluated kidney biopsies of living and deceased patients for the presence of viral protein by immunohistology, immunofluorescence, viral RNA by in situ hybridization, or viral RNA polymerase chair reaction (PCR) testing and found that 43% of patients had sars-coV-2 infection present. Subsequent studies have detected sars-coV-2 RNA with viral replication occurring in the tubular epithelial cells of the kidneys in 73% of patients with sars-coV-2 infection and AKI.[13] Urine testing for sars-coV-2 RNA has also been conducted and was present less frequently in the urine (8%) when compared with blood (21%) and stool (40%) when compared in a meta-analysis of 30 studies.[9] Some theorize that the alteration or dysregulation of the immune system is related to uremic syndrome in patients with ESRD or due to the effects of immunosuppressive medications after transplantation and is attributed to the variability noted in susceptibility, course, and severity of illness, and subsequently outcomes.[14,15]

The prevalence of sars-coV-2 infection among patients with CKD in the United States varies depending on the study with rates ranging from 3.5% to 48%.[8] A large cohort study conducted by Pakhchanian and colleagues (2021) concluded that the presence of CKD is an independent risk factor for severe sars-coV-2 infection. A patient's risk heightens with the presence of additional comorbid conditions. Patients with CKD stage 3 and sars-coV-2 infection have a higher risk for requiring renal replacement therapy.[13] An observational, retrospective study (n = 3905) was conducted by Kharti and colleagues (2021) and evaluated the health outcomes of individuals with sars-coV-2 infection and CKD or ESRD, and without CKD. Mortality rates were higher for individuals with kidney disease. Early in the COVID-19 pandemic, the overall rate of mortality for individuals with CKD was 34% and 27% for individuals with ESRD requiring dialysis.[7] The overall mortality for individuals without kidney disease was 24%.[7] The highest rate of mortality was among individuals with sars-coV-2 infection and CKD.[7]

Renal transplant patients have been one of the populations most vulnerable to sars-coV-2 infection. The number of kidney transplants performed from 2020 (n = 22,817) to 2021 (n = 24,670) increased 8.14%.[16] In this pandemic era, management of induction and maintenance immunosuppression has been challenging to clinicians treating kidney transplant patients. COVID-19 has had a significant influence on wait-listed patients, elucidating the need to properly balance the risks and benefits of transplantation in the setting of an ongoing pandemic.

CHALLENGES ENCOUNTERED

There have been multiple challenges experienced during the COVID-19 pandemic with lessons learned for future pandemics, public health emergencies, or disasters. Unclear messaging regarding the COVID-19 from public health officials created challenges for health-care providers and patients resulting in the lack of preparedness and timely response due to the uncertainty of the virus. Diagnostic, treatment, logistical, and preventive challenges were identified during the delivery of care to patients with kidney disease during the COVID-19 pandemic. Gaps in planning efforts were identified that led to challenges affecting the availability of staff, infection control measures, and allocation of resources.

Clinical Presentation

Clinical presentation depends on organ involvement, severity of disease, and individual patient factors. The clinical presentation of sars-coV-2 infection in individuals with kidney disease presented unique challenges. The classic symptoms of sars-coV-2 infection reported from the general population included fever, cough, lack of taste, and/or smell. Early studies demonstrated that the clinical presentation of sars-coV-2 infection in patients with ESRD receiving dialysis was atypical and varied from the general population. Individuals with ESRD and the early stage of sars-coV-2 infection presented with symptoms commonly associated with uremia such as fatigue and anorexia making the diagnosis of COVID-19 challenging. Respiratory symptoms, fever, and lymphadenopathy were experienced less frequently among individuals with ESRD and sars-coV-2 infection. The lack of fever and cough in the ESRD population raised questions regarding the generalizability of the data from the general population.[7] The atypical response may reflect an altered immune response and ability to mount the characteristic cytokine storm.[7] Although the ESRD population often experiences less symptoms at the onset of the disease, the clinical course of the disease was frequently characterized by more severity of disease, higher rates of bilateral lung fields affected, complications such as shock, acute respiratory distress syndrome, myocardial infarction, arrhythmias, and death than the general population (14% vs 4%) demonstrating the need for an increased vigilance.[5,17] It is imperative that nurses are aware of the potential atypical presentations of sars-coV-2 infection in individuals with kidney disease for an early identification and treatment.

Treatment Challenges

A patient with sars-coV-2 infection was at a 130% increased risk for the development of AKI during the pandemic compared with prepandemic.[18] Treatment of AKI in hemodynamically unstable patients includes supportive therapy and the use of CRRT. Anger and colleagues (2021) studied the demand for CRRT equipment and supplies during the pandemic comparing prepandemic use from a manufacturer's perspective. The use of CRRT increased 370% with a shortage of 1088 CRRT machines within the first 6 months of the pandemic.[18] By the peak of the pandemic, the number of CRRT machines used increased by 279%.[18] The demand for dialysis fluids also increased significantly causing an increased need for production and approval of an emergency use order, which permitted the use of fluids imported from other countries.[18] Some hospitals were forced to produce their own fluids due to the shortage.[18] To increase production at the manufacturing company, protocols to ensure the safety of the employees had to be developed. Manufacturing had to be increased and protocols reevaluated to streamline distribution. Training of the employees and troubleshooting services for the nurses had to be converted to a virtual environment, which increased staff training by 300%.[18] Important lessons learned include continued maintenance of emergency preparedness plans is essential to ensure the continuity of operations; refurbished machines can be held in reserve to use if needed; inventory and patient census should be closely monitored; and an inventory management system to include tracking should be developed or improved.[18]

Infection Control Measures

Controlling the spread of sars-coV-2 infection in the dialysis facilities presented a multitude of unique challenges further challenging current infection control measures. The primary focus of prior infection control efforts included suppressing the transmission of blood-borne infections. Transmission of a highly contagious airborne disease that caused a worldwide pandemic was not anticipated. Because the COVID-19 pandemic evolved, additional logistical challenges emerged. Individuals with ESRD and receiving hemodialysis as well as the clinic staff were unable to comply with the stay-at-home orders during the COVID-19 pandemic, which contributed to a higher risk for contracting the sars-coV-2 infection due to repeated and prolonged exposure. In some instances, the infection spread among the patients and the clinic's staff causing clustering of cases.[17] To reduce the cluster outbreaks and the rapid respiratory transmission of the sars-coV-2 infection, dialysis facilities implemented universal respiratory precautions such as screening for symptoms and temperature screenings on entry into the facilities, masking during treatment, additional handwashing, and distancing to reduce the spread. The number of provider rounds conducted in person was limited and visits transitioned to a virtual telehealth format. The number of patients receiving treatment during a shift was also limited to assist with reducing exposure.[8] Limiting the number of patients per shift may extend the number of hours that the nurses and clinic staff worked, which could lead to exhaustion and burnout.

Most dialysis units are designed with patients seated more than 6 feet apart, which has been a benefit for complying with the social distancing requirements. Depending on the method of transportation that the patient utilized, social distancing may have been difficult to maintain during transportation.[17] Each dialysis clinic has at least one isolation room that may be available for isolating patients with suspected sars-coV-2 infection as needed. However, the need for isolation quickly exceeded the availability, leading to the need for designated COVID-19 units or shifts to be created. Logistical challenges were encountered with the creation of the designated COVID-19 units or shifts. Ideally, a dialysis clinic is close to a patient's home. Transportation to the clinic is usually by the patient, family, friends, or a hired service. The parish or county that a patient resides in often offers public transportation services for medical visits. The location of the designated COVID-19 units presented unique transportation challenges especially if travel across parish lines was required and often created access barriers. Public transportation services for medical visits do not offer travel across parish lines.

Because COVID-19 testing efforts expanded, there were many patients that tested positive for sars-coV-2 infection but were asymptomatic, which created complex decisions about the most appropriate isolation method for these individuals. According to a study conducted by Kharti and colleagues (2021), approximately 32% of all COVID-19 cases in the outpatient dialysis clinics were asymptomatic. Prevalence rates were variable among units depending on the comorbid conditions, age, and other vulnerabilities of the population.[7] Evidence is currently lacking regarding the asymptomatic transmission among vulnerable individuals.[7] Additional questions surrounded when an individual could safely return to the dialysis clinic following recovery from sars-coV-2 infection and no longer transmit the virus to others in the clinic. Until formalized guidance was developed, decisions were determined on a case-by-case basis. Because the COVID-19 pandemic continued to unfold, The Centers for Disease Control (CDC) and Prevention (2021) developed recommendations that included 2 negative test results within a 24-hour period, the onset of symptoms was more than 14 days ago, and that the patient was afebrile for more than 72 hours.[8] Another challenge encountered included patients that persistently tested positive but were asymptomatic. The CDC determined that patients who are asymptomatic could no longer transmit the virus after 10 days.[17] For patients who are immunocompromised or have severe disease, the recommendation is 20 days before returning to the clinic.[17] Additional research is needed to identify how long an asymptomatic patient receiving dialysis can transmit live virus after recovering from sars-coV-2 infection.[17] Many argue that individuals with ESRD and receiving dialysis should be considered immunocompromised, which further complicates the decision of whether 10 or 20 days is most appropriate. Thus, more research is needed.

Supply Chain Problems

The COVID-19 pandemic caused immense disruption to the dialysis equipment supply chain. Similar to the limited number of ventilators during the initial surge of sars-coV-2 cases, dialysis machines, other dialysis-related equipment, personnel, and personal protective gear were also in short supply. When the demand for treatment exceeds the supply of personnel and equipment necessary to administer dialysis, providers are called on for complex ethical decision-making. With the COVID-19 pandemic, patients with AKI requiring dialysis were admitted to the intensive care units overwhelming the current system and allocation of resources.[18] The preparation for pandemics or other large-scale disasters should be part of disaster planning and include efforts addressing dialysis needs. Allocation of resources should include consideration of surge capacity, outpatient and inpatient dialysis needs for future pandemic and/or disaster needs. Distribution of resources should be adequate and ethical. The medical community has often placed the focus on optimizing the aggregate benefit. Carson and colleagues (2021) in Canada proposed an ethical framework for the allocation of dialysis services to reduce distress associated with decision-making and to optimize decision-making utilizing the framework. The ethical principles utilized to create this framework include maximizing benefits, equitable treatment of individuals, prioritizing the individuals who are more severe, and procedural justice.[18]

Vaccination

Kidney disease also affects the effectiveness of vaccination. Several barriers have been identified. Initial drug trials often exclude individuals with kidney disease, thus there are limited data available regarding vaccine effectiveness. Because kidney function declines, an individual's response to a vaccination is altered.[19–24] Hepatitis B and Influenza A vaccines have been studied to identify alternative strategies for improving responsiveness to vaccines for individuals with kidney disease.[19] The COVID-19 vaccinations developed also excluded individuals on dialysis, limiting the data available regarding humoral and cellular response among the dialysis population.[19] Before the study conducted by Speer and colleagues[19] (2021), varying results of seroconversion were noted in smaller studies. Methods to ensure success of vaccination for individuals with kidney disease and at a higher risk for contracting sars-coV-2 infection are crucial. Additionally, vaccination protocols may require different protocols depending on degree of kidney function. Speers and colleagues, (2021) conducted a prospective, single center study, which was one of the earliest studies evaluating the humoral response of individuals receiving dialysis after vaccination with the BioNTech 162b2 mRNA vaccine. Individuals receiving dialysis (n = 22) were compared with healthy individuals without CKD (n = 46). Antibody levels were measured before enrollment and following vaccinations. Antigen rapid tests for sars-coV-2 infection were performed before each dialysis treatment. Individuals that contracted the disease were excluded. IgG levels were also monitored. Due to the difference in age among the dialysis and control groups, a subanalysis was performed. Speers and colleagues (2021) identified that individuals on dialysis developed significantly less sars-coV-2 anti-S1 IgG antibodies following the first and second COVID-19 vaccination compared with the age-matched healthy individuals. The results obtained by Speers and colleagues (2021) were consistent with prior studies examining the immune response of individuals receiving the influenza A and Hepatitis B vaccines in the presence of kidney disease. Individuals receiving dialysis are a high-risk group for sars-coV-2 infection. The findings by Speer and colleagues[19] (2021) indicate that the first COVID-19 vaccination dose may not provide adequate coverage. Additional research is needed to evaluate the response and effectiveness of vaccinations for individuals receiving dialysis.

NURSING IMPLICATIONS

The challenges encountered during the COVID-19 pandemic have presented valuable lessons learned for future pandemics, other public health emergencies, and disasters. Emergent disease such as COVID-19 created crisis in the health-care system and challenged existing roles. Organizational priorities and staff responsibilities shifted. Nursing leadership is critical during health-care challenges that cause widespread disruption to the delivery of health care. The COVID-19 pandemic has further exposed the extensive need for more nurses to be knowledgeable about the care of kidney disease and receive the specialized training required to administer dialysis effectively. The significant increase in the need for dialysis nursing services also reinforced the realization that the shortage of dialysis nurses needs to be addressed. The patient advocacy role of nephrology nurses is vital, allowing the nurse to assist patients in gaining a full understanding of their treatment plan and participate in decision-making. Incorporating education to increase patient awareness, methods for prevention and to reduce the progression of disease, the complications of CKD, dialysis modalities, and dialysis management into nursing education could increase interest in nephrology nursing and reduce the nursing shortages in nephrology.

Multiple areas for improvement at the institutional and systems level were unveiled. Planning efforts should include preparation for pandemics or other large-scale disasters. Targeted training, drills, and exercises should be executed to assist in preparedness for readiness to respond. Nursing's involvement in improving health and health care for all patients at a policy level is but an extension of the advocacy work. Facility-level policies are needed to reduce the spread of an infectious disease in a congregate setting such as the dialysis facilities, universal infection control measures that address multiple routes of transmission, methods to isolate patients when test results are pending, infection control measures when delivering a dialysis treatment to a patient who is in isolation while protecting the nurse from exposure, and the increased use of personal protective equipment. Policies limiting access to health care related to medical transportation across parish/county lines during times of disaster or a pandemic need to be reevaluated and barriers eliminated. Policies at the system and facility levels to address the development of ethical, evidence-based methods for allocating resources during times when the need for resources significantly exceeds the supply. Allocation of resources should include consideration of surge capacity, outpatient and inpatient dialysis needs for future pandemic and/or disaster needs. Distribution of resources should be adequate, equitable as possible, and ethical.

The COVID-19 pandemic is occurring within a context of social and economic inequalities. Inequalities in COVID-19 infection and mortality rates are a result of inequalities in chronic diseases such as renal disease and are socially patterned and associated with the social determinants of health. Nurses can be strategic contributors to making substantive progress toward achieving health-care equity by taking on expanded roles, working in innovative ways, and partnering with communities and other sectors.

Nursing implications for research include that additional research is needed regarding the best methods for vaccination of individuals with kidney disease. The best methods for infection control in a congregate setting also require additional research.

SUMMARY

The COVID-19 pandemic disproportionately affected individuals with kidney disease causing significant morbidity and mortality worldwide. Sars-coV-2 infection has been linked to the development of AKI and worsening of underlying kidney function. The long-term sequelae of sars-coV-2 infection and kidney disease remain to be seen. System, provider, and patient level challenges have been identified during the COVID-19 pandemic. Nurses are the largest group of health-care professionals in the United States and must be knowledgeable regarding the care of individuals with kidney disease. Nursing leaders are needed to identify innovative methods for educating the nursing workforce that is specialized in nephrology care, reduce the nephrology nursing shortage, to address the diagnostic, treatment, logistical, and preventive challenges identified, and to improve the delivery of nephrology health care.

CLINICS CARE POINTS

- Approximately 90% of individuals with kidney disease lack awareness of their disease status which contributes to poor health outcomes due to missed opportunities for treatment and prevention.
- Clinical Practice Guidelines for the care of individuals with kidney disease are available from the National Kidney Foundation KDOQI at https://kidney.org/professionals/guidelines and from Kidney Disease Improving Global Outcomes (KDIGO) at https://kdigo.org/guidelines/.

DISCLOSURE

The authors have nothing to disclose.

REFERENCES

1. National Kidney Foundation. NKF and optumlabs call for changes to improve kidney health. 2021. Available at. https://www.kidney.org/news/nkf-and-optumlabs-call-changes-to-improve-kidney-health. Accessed June 1, 2022.
2. United States Renal Data System (USRDS). Annual data report. 2021. Available at. https://adr.usrds.org/2021. Accessed June 1, 2022.
3. USRDS. Annual data report. 2020. Available at. https://adr.usrds.org/2020/. Accessed June 1, 2022.
4. Boyle SM, Washington R, McCann P, et al. The nephrology nursing shortage: insights from a pandemic. Am J Kidney Dis 2022;79(1):113–6.
5. Ajaimy M, Melamed ML. COVID-19 in patients with kidney disease. Clin J Am Soc Nephrolrol 2020;15:1087–9.
6. Palevsky PM. COVID-19 and AKI: where do we stand? J Am Soc Nephrolrol 2021; 32:1029–32.
7. Kharti M, Islam S, Dutka P, et al. COVID-19 antibodies and outcomes among outpatient maintenance hemodialysis patients. Kidney 2021;360(2):263–9.
8. McAdams M, Ostrosky-Frid M, Rajora N, et al. Effect of COVID-19 on kidney disease incidence and management. Kidney 2021;360(2):141–53.
9. Hassler L, Reyes F, Sparks M, et al. Evidence for and against direct kidney infection by Sars-Cov-2 in patients with COVID-19. Clin J Am Soc Nephrol 2021;16: 1755–65.
10. Scherer JS, Qian Y, Rau ME, et al. Utilization of palliative care for patients and covid-19 infection and acute kidney injury during a COVID-19 surge. Clin J Am Soc Nephrol 2022;17:342–9.

11. Moledina D, Simonov M, Yamamoto Y, et al. The association of COVID-19 with acute kidney injury independent of severity of illness: a multicenter cohort study. Am J Kidney Dis 2021;77(4):490–9.e1.
12. Chan L, Chaudhary K, Saha A, et al. AKI in hospitalized patients with COVID-19. J Am Soc Nephrol 2021;32:151–60.
13. Karras A, Livrozet M, Lazareth H, et al. Proteinuria and clinical outcomes in hospitalized COVID-19 patients: a retrospective single-center study. Clin J Am Soc Nephrol 2021;16:514–21.
14. De Meester J, De Bacquer D, Naesens M, et al. Incidence, characteristics, and outcome of COVID-19 in adults on kidney replacement therapy: a regionwide registry study. J Am Soc Nephrol 2021;32:385–96.
15. Pakhchanian H, Raiker R, Mukherjee A, et al. Outcomes of COVID-19 in CKD patients: a multicenter electronic medical record cohort study. Clin J Am Soc Nephrol 2021;16:785–6.
16. Organ Procurement & Transplant Network. National transplant data. Available at. https://optn.transplant.hrsa.gov/data/view-data-reports/national-data/. Accessed June 1, 2022.
17. Wu J, Zhu G, Zhang Y, et al. Clinical features of maintenance hemodialysis patients with 2019 novel coronavirus-infected pneumonia in Wuhan, China. Clin J Am Soc Nephrol 2019;15:1139–45.
18. Anger MS, Mullon C, Ficociello LH, et al. Meeting the demand for renal replacment therapy during the COVID-19 pandemic: a manufacturer's perspective. Kidney 2021;360(2):350–4.
19. Kliger AS, Silberzweig J. COVID-19 and dialysis patients: unsolved problems in early 2021. J Am Soc Nephrol 2021;32:1018–20.
20. Carson RC, Forzley B, Thomas S, et al. Balancing the needs of acute and maintenancE PATIENTS DUring the COVID-19 pandemic: a proposed ethical framework for dialysis allocation. Clin J Am Soc Nephrol 2021;16:1122–30.
21. Speer C, Goth D, Benning L, et al. Early humoral responses of hemodialysis patients after COVID-19 vaccination with BNT162b2. Clin J Am Soc Nephrol 2021;16:1073–82.
22. Butler CR, Wightman AG. Scare health care resources and equity during COVID-19: lessons from the history of kidney failure treatment. Kidney 2021;360(2):2024–6.
23. Craig-Schapiro R, Salinas T, Lubetzky M, et al. COVID-19 outcomes in patients waitlisted for kidney transplantation and kidney transplant recipients. Am J Transplant 2021;21(4):1576–85.
24. Srivatana V, Wilkies C, Perl J, et al. Vaccine and the need to be heard: considerations for COVID-19 immunization in ESKD. Kidney 2021;360(2):1048–50.

Transitions of Care Considerations for Nephrology Patients

Sherry Rivera, DNP, APRN, ANP-C, FNKF[a],*,
Lyn Behnke, DNP, FNP-BCBC, PMHNP-BC, CAFCI, CHFN[b],
M.J. Henderson, MS, RN, GNP-BC (retired)[c]

KEYWORDS

- Kidney disease • Transitions of care • Older adults • Acute kidney injury
- Transitional care

KEY POINTS

- Kidney disease is a significant health problem and affects 10% of the population world-wide and 15% of the population in the United States.
- Acute kidney injury is a growing global issue and continues to present significant risk to the older adult population.
- Nurses are critical to a successful transition of care.
- Individuals with kidney disease have multiple underlying comorbid conditions and encounter many transitions of care placing them at higher risk for adverse events to occur.

INTRODUCTION

According to the Administration on Aging (2021), almost 22% of the population in the United States will be composed of adults over the age of 65 years by the year 2040. It is anticipated that the population of older adults will reach 94.7 million people by 2060.[1] The need for a workforce able to address the health care needs of older adults has been well established. Nurses will have a vital role in providing care to older adults and addressing the societal challenges that present with the growth in the population. Complicating matters further, the expansion of the nursing shortage coincides with the anticipated growth of the older adult population. According to the American Association of Colleges of Nursing (AACN, 2020), the shortage of nurses is projected to increase between 2016 and 2030.[2] In 2010, *The Future of Nursing* called for an increase in the number of baccalaureate prepared nurses to 80% and doubling the

[a] Nurse Practitioner Program, Louisiana State University Health New Orleans School of Nursing, 1900 Gravier Street, New Orleans, LA 70112, USA; [b] University of Michigan-Flint, School of Nursing; [c] Gerontological Nurse Consultant
* Corresponding author.
E-mail address: Srive4@lsuhsc.edu

Crit Care Nurs Clin N Am 34 (2022) 491–500
https://doi.org/10.1016/j.cnc.2022.07.006
0899-5885/22/© 2022 Elsevier Inc. All rights reserved.

number of nurses with doctoral degrees to address the health care needs of the older adult population.[2] The Institute of Medicine workforce target goals as described by the AACN remain unmet.[3] According to the latest release of the *Future of Nursing 2020 to 2030*, the nursing profession will be challenged to care for an aging population with multiple complex comorbid conditions.[4] Comorbid conditions are prevalent among older adults in America with 51.8% having at least one comorbid condition and 27.2% having two or more comorbid conditions.[1,5] Given the complexity of illness and the growing numbers of the older adult population along with the continued shortage of nurses, it is imperative that nurses and nurse practitioners (NPs) are prepared to address the complex health care needs of an older adult population.

Older Adults and Kidney Disease

Kidney disease is a significant health problem and affects 10% of the population worldwide and 15% of the population in the United States.[6] Advanced age and/or the presence of comorbid conditions increases the prevalence of kidney disease.[7] According to the United States Renal Data System (USRDS. 2021), the prevalence of chronic kidney disease (CKD) increased from 8.0% in 2009 to 14.2% in 2019 among Medicare recipients ages 66 years or older.[7] For individuals 85 years of age and older the prevalence of CKD is 23.9%.[8] Annually, kidney disease accounts for over 120 billion dollars of the Medicare budget.[8] Over 50% of the individuals receiving dialysis are over the age of 65 years.[8] An individual who is 65 years of age or older has twice the rate of mortality risk than those of the general population who have diabetes, cancer, heart failure, cerebrovascular accident, or an acute myocardial infarction.[8] Up until the COVID-19 pandemic, the number of individuals with end-stage renal disease (ESRD) requiring dialysis was rising.[8] For the first time, the number of individuals with ESRD decreased most likely due to the number of deaths related to sars-coV-2 infection among the dialysis population.[9]

Risk factors for the development of kidney disease includes the normal aging process, age-related changes in volume status, lack of provider and patient awareness, medications, hypertension, diabetes mellitus, and other comorbid conditions that can heighten the risk for development of acute kidney injury (AKI) and/or progression of CKD. Complicating matters further, older adults may be exposed to multiple nephrotoxic medications during hospitalization. The percentage of AKI related to medication in the older adult population varies between 14% and 26% depending on the source cited. Older adults may have a decreased renal reserve making it difficult for them to mount an appropriate compensatory mechanism when under periods of stress related to illness which heightens their risk for developing AKI. Worsening kidney function increases the rates of morbidity and mortality. By age 75 years, more than 50% of older adults have developed kidney disease which may be related to the aging process, underlying risk factors, and/or comorbid conditions.[6] The percentage of individuals who have acquired kidney disease related to sars-coV-2 infection and the long-term sequela remain to be seen.

AKI is a growing global issue and continues to present significant risk to the older adult population. Diagnosis of AKI has been improving due to heightened awareness and better detection. The rate of first-time hospitalizations with AKI in the older adult population has increased by 42% since 2009 with rates of admissions increasing with advancing age.[7] For adults ages 75 to 84 years, there were 60.0 admissions per 1000 person-years and 115.9 admissions per 1000 person-years for adults of 85 years of age or older.[7] Admission rates also vary by race with Medicare beneficiaries who are black (87.2 admissions per 1000 person years) which is a 67% higher rate than Medicare beneficiaries who are white.[7] The development of AKI can contribute to a higher rate for subsequent episodes of AKI, readmission to the hospital within 1 to 2 years, and a higher risk for death within the same time frame. According to the USRDS (2021), approximately 27% of older adults are readmitted to the hospital within 1 year and 35.1% will be readmitted within 2 years following an episode of AKI. The presence of underlying comorbid conditions such as diabetes and CKD has a seven times higher risk for developing AKI.[7] Individuals with AKI were also more likely to die within the first 2 years following discharge from the hospital (30.9% at 1 year and 41.2% at 2 years).[7]

Survivors of AKI are at an increased risk for progression of kidney disease. According to Silver and Siew,[10] AKI survivors are ten times more likely to have progressive CKD, three times higher risk for ESRD, and two times higher risk for death. The risk for progression from AKI to CKD and ESRD is highest among the older adult population.[11] Individuals who are 67 years of age or older with AKI and underlying CKD have 41 times higher risk for developing ESRD.[11] Among individuals requiring dialysis during hospitalization for AKI, 12.9% were diagnosed with ESRD within 1 month of discharge, and 17.7% within 6 months following discharge.[7] A lack of referral to nephrology or delayed referral can result in delayed diagnosis and may result in progression of disease. Some studies demonstrate that decreased mortality rates are associated with earlier referral rates to nephrology.[11]

Overall, a diagnosis of kidney disease corresponds to higher rates of emergency department visits, hospitalizations, and mortality rates especially for the older adult population. The rates of hospitalization and mortality are twice as high among individuals with kidney disease than individuals without kidney disease.[7] Worsening kidney function to the advanced stages of disease also corresponds to a rise in the number of hospitalizations. Prior to the COVID-19 pandemic, one in five individuals discharged from the hospital with CKD were readmitted within 30 days.[7] In addition, one in fifteen individuals with CKD died following discharge.[7] To prevent readmissions and deaths following discharge, improvement in post discharge care is needed. Given the number of providers and facilities involved, medications, and complexities of care, it is imperative that the appropriate information is communicated, and that care is coordinated. Nurses and nurse practitioners have a vitally important role for ensuring communication and the coordination of care to improve the health outcomes of the older adult with kidney disease.

Evidence-Based Guidelines for Safe Transitions of Care

Nurses are critical to a successful transition of care. Nurses who are familiar with strategies to use when assisting older adults during the transitions of care are essential. Naylor's Transitional Care Model is an evidence-based, nurse-led, team-based model used to improve the quality of care for individuals and families while reducing health care costs as during transitions across multiple settings and providers.[12] Identification of the individual's health care goals is a vital component when determining the plan of care. Communication between nurses and NPs can ensure consistent delivery of the plan of care. The nine components of the model include screening, staffing, maintaining relationships, engaging patients and families or caregivers, assessing/managing risks, and symptoms, educating/promoting self-management, collaborating, promoting continuity, and fostering coordination.[12] Screening should include identification of individuals who are at a higher risk for poor outcomes. Some key risk factors that would heighten a nurse's concern for poor outcomes would include individuals with five or more active chronic conditions, history of a recent fall, difficulty with the activities of daily living, presence of dementia or other cognitive impairment, history of mental health challenges, age, lack of support, and prior hospitalization within the last 30 days or more than two hospitalizations within the last six months.[12] Nurse practitioners establish and maintain a therapeutic, trusting relationship with the individual and their families/caregivers, promote continuity, and collaborate with other providers to ensure high-quality care across the transitions of care.

Transitions of Care

There are primarily two types of transitions of care that can occur for individuals with kidney disease. The first involves the multiple transitions that can occur across multiple health care settings and providers. The most common transition is from hospital to home or vice versa. Individuals with kidney disease have multiple providers involved in their care and complex treatment regimens involving numerous medications and dietary changes creating the potential for errors to occur. The second type of transition that has recently been discussed in literature is related to the transitions that an individual encounters related to the complexities of care such as the transitions of diagnosis, complex treatment regimens, dialysis, transitions between types of dialysis, transplantation, and conservative care. In addition to coping with a new diagnosis of kidney disease, transition to an outpatient dialysis clinic causes drastic changes to an individual's lifestyle, diet, daily routine, placement of a long-term vascular access, and adds multiple health care providers to the care team. Individuals in the acute care setting may transition quickly through the stages of transitions making adaptation difficult and complex. An individual's risk for death is higher within the first 6 months of transitioning to dialysis or transplantation.[13] Depending on the individual's functional status following hospitalization, some individuals may also require transition to a skilled nursing facility. Individuals with kidney disease experience a significant number of transitions of care throughout their life and the course of their disease. Owing to the complexities in management of kidney disease, the transitions of care may be poorly managed resulting in an increased risk for errors.

Current literature has described the need for consideration of transition clinics to better prepare individuals with kidney disease for dialysis, transplantation, or conservative care. Referral to nephrology 3 to 6 months before initiation of renal replacement therapy is associated with improved outcomes, lower rates of hospitalization, improved access to peritoneal dialysis and transplantation waitlists, lower rates of initiation of renal replacement therapy, and central venous catheters.[14] The Kidney Disease Improving Global Outcomes (KDIGO) recommends individuals with progression of CKD, an estimated glomerular filtration rate (eGFR) less than 30 mL/min, and the presence of albuminuria greater than 30 mg/mmol be referred to nephrology.[15] Kidney disease-related transitions of care should include patient education, advanced care planning, and discussions about dialysis modalities, vascular access, conservative medical management, and transplantation options. The USRDS Transition of Care in Chronic Kidney Disease has been monitoring the mortality rates of individuals who transition to dialysis.[8] Additional research is needed to determine the optimal timing for initiating dialysis to improve outcomes.

Individuals with complex health care needs use more health care services thus increasing the number of transitions of care that a patient encounters. Individuals with CKD have multiple underlying comorbid conditions and encounter many transitions of care across multiple settings with numerous providers placing them at a higher risk for adverse events to occur. An individual with CKD has an average of seven providers by CKD stages 4 and 12 providers by CKD stage 5.[16] The average number of specialists increases as well. Individuals with stage 4 CKD have an average of 10 specialists and an average of 16 specialists by CKD stage 5. The number of health care encounters increases with the advancing stages of kidney disease. Each transition of care increases the risk for medication errors and quality or safety problems.[16] Communication and continuity of care are required during every transition of care. Providers need to be knowledgeable regarding the complexity of CKD management and potential for miscommunication. Primary care providers are vitally important for coordinating care and communicating between specialists. Communication and collaboration are essential for the delivery of high-quality care. Providers and individuals with CKD must be able to communicate with multiple providers across multiple settings to ensure high quality appropriate care is delivered.

Decisions to be considered for post hospital follow up include, timing of follow-up, provider type for follow up (primary care provider vs nephrologist), coordination of care for various medical services depending on the needs of the individual, outpatient dialysis treatments, and communication with other providers and specialists. The timing of follow up depends on the severity of AKI experienced, comorbid conditions present, recovery of kidney function, dialysis dependence, and whether the individual was discharged to home or transferred to a long-term facility. Nephrologist input regarding the timing of follow-up post hospitalization is a valuable resource.

Current literature has varying recommendations regarding post hospitalization follow-up. According to the USRDS, only 28.9% of survivors of AKI requiring dialysis followed up with nephrology within 6 months of discharge, whereas only 7.9% of those who did not require dialysis saw a nephrologist.[7] Harel and colleagues noted that individuals who followed up with nephrology within 90 days of discharge following a severe episode of AKI requiring dialysis had a lower 2-year mortality rate than those who did not follow up with nephrology.[17] The 15th Acute Dialysis Quality Initiative Consensus Statement (2016) recommends that hospital systems develop a structure and process for improving the documentation of an episode of AKI, monitoring measures to track short- and long-term outcomes following an episode of AKI, and recommendations for post hospitalization follow-up visits.[18] The KDIGO AKI Clinical Practice Guidelines (2012) recommend that at a minimum individuals should be reevaluated within 3 months following an episode of AKI to determine whether kidney function has improved or progressed.[15] Determination of an individual's risk factors, etiology of onset, and severity of the AKI episode should be considered for follow-up instructions and monitoring. Patients who have not regained kidney function and continue to require dialysis will be seen in the outpatient dialysis setting. Patients with partially regained kidney function may require follow up within 1 to 2 weeks depending on severity. Individuals with fully regained kidney function and less severe kidney disease may not require follow up for several weeks. It is imperative that patients are not lost to follow up due to the higher risk for a subsequent episode of AKI, rehospitalization, and death. Clinicians evaluating kidney function using a basic or comprehensive metabolic panel including an eGFR and urine studies to evaluate proteinuria (urine albumin to creatinine ratio or urine protein to creatinine ratio) should do so before discharge to provide valuable information for comparison post hospitalization. According to the USRDS (2020), only 76.3% of individuals have kidney function testing within 6 months of discharge after an episode of AKI.[19] Hospital discharge summaries should include AKI diagnoses, etiology, and hospital course. A retrospective chart review conducted by Greer and colleagues revealed that only 44% of charts included documentation of an AKI diagnosis with only 43% listing etiology and 31% including the hospital course.[17] Specific instructions were only included 13% of the time and 6% included follow-up plans.[17] Improvement is needed to improve the outcomes of individuals experiencing AKI. Nurses and nurse practitioners must be knowledgeable regarding the risks, recommendations, and complexity of care required for the older adult experiencing an episode of AKI. Communication among all providers, and facilities providing health care services is vital to ensure coordination of care and delivery of high-quality consistent care.

Polypharmacy

Polypharmacy is also a contributing factor for adverse events in all settings and patient populations. Polypharmacy occurs in 80% of individuals with CKD.[14] Medication reconciliation is a key aspect of transitional care and involves more than just obtaining a list of current medications from an individual or medical records. When conducting a medication reconciliation, it should be in-depth and include the indication for use, appropriate monitoring, or testing. Prescribed, over the counter medications, dietary supplements, and vitamins can heighten the risk for interactions and exposure to nephrotoxic medications in the older adult population with kidney disease and complex conditions. An individual with CKD takes an average of 6 to 12 medications. An individual with ESRD consumes an average of 19 pills per day with 25% of this population using more than 25 medications daily.[20] Medication reconciliation should also include a review of potentially nephrotoxic medications and be reevaluated with changes in an individual's kidney function. AKI can occur during hospitalization due to potentially nephrotoxic agents such as intravenous (IV) contrast dye, nonsteroidal anti-inflammatory medications, diuretics, angiotensin-converting enzyme inhibitors, angiotensin II blockers, antibiotics, and other medications.

Older adults at a higher risk for readmission and poor outcomes during transitions of care.[21] Poor communication is the most common cause of errors that occur during the transitions of care and a contributing factor for hospital readmissions.[3,22] Older adults with kidney disease are especially vulnerable requiring extensive coordination of care and communication. The discharge summary often serves as the primary source for communication. Direct communication is vitally important for communicating information that may require close monitoring and follow up.[21] Methods to improve communication, via the availability of discharge summaries in the early discharge period, and follow up with a primary care provider within a month of discharge has been linked to a reduction in hospital readmissions.[23] The discharge documentation for older adult patients should include documentation of a patient's functional level, cognitive ability, and advanced care planning preferences.[21] Standardization of data collection methods facilitates improving rates of documentation of quality indicators and reduced rates of mortality within a year following discharge.[24] To ensure a positive patient experience, it is important to provide explanations of the current situation, confirm understanding of the situation, and discuss future steps. By incorporating patient preferences and empowering patients and their families to be active participants in their care will facilitate delivery of patient centered care.

Case Study

Phyllis is a 77-year-old woman who was admitted for a chief complaint of shortness of breath and dyspnea on exertion. She uses 2 L of oxygen via nasal cannula at home and was noted to be hypoxemic with an oxygen saturation of 66%. She was seen by her primary care provider who recommended transfer to the tertiary care hospital via ambulance because she was hypoxemic with an oxygen saturation of 66%. Phyllis resides in a rural area, so the closest tertiary care hospital is located 2 hours away. Owing to the cost of ambulance transport, Phyllis refused. Despite NP recommendations, Phyllis's son began driving his mother to the hospital. Unfortunately, after about an hour of driving, Phyllis' mental status declined requiring her son to stop at a community hospital. Phyllis was then transferred via ambulance to the tertiary care hospital.

Upon admission to the tertiary hospital, she was intubated and admitted to the intensive care unit where she was diagnosed with pneumonia and an acute exacerbation of chronic obstructive pulmonary disease (COPD). She was started on a broad-spectrum antibiotic and steroids. After 7 days of no improvement and a negative COVID test, she was given IV diuretics and her code status changed to do not resuscitate. She responded well to diuresis, but her blood urea nitrogen and serum creatinine remained elevated, and nephrology was consulted for evaluation of AKI. Continuous renal replacement therapy was initiated due to metabolic acidosis, azotemia, fluid overload, and oliguria. Over the course of hospitalization, she was transitioned to intermittent hemodialysis. A tunneled dialysis catheter was inserted into her right internal jugular vein as access for dialysis. Phyllis was extubated on day 8 of admission. An echocardiogram was obtained and showed an ejection fraction of 69% with both right ventricular hypertrophy and left ventricular hypertrophy.

Phyllis continued to improve over the course of the admission and was discharged home on the 14th day. She refused admission to a skilled nursing facility. Her baseline medical history included COPD, opioid addiction, hypertension, obesity, osteoarthritis of the back and hips, chronic pain, deconditioning, CKD, and diabetes type 2. Her last hemoglobin A1C was 7.0%. Past surgical history included hysterectomy at the age of 30 years and four back surgeries with the most recent one in 2019. She became addicted to opioid pain medication with her most recent back surgery but has continued to comply with a treatment program. Several safety challenges were identified when evaluating her housing situation and respiratory condition. She was constantly exposed to methamphetamine in her apartment building which caused her to use her rescue inhaler more frequently. There was also mold from some water damage that had not yet been repaired. She worked as a housekeeper for many years and was paid cash so is ineligible for social security but has Medicaid.

Her discharge diagnoses were the same as her pre-admission diagnoses except for AKI which did not resolve before discharge. She was referred to an outpatient dialysis clinic for continued hemodialysis treatments. Medications at discharge included fluticasone furoate 100 mcg and vilanterol 25 mcg inhalation powder 2 puffs daily, lisinopril 20 mg daily, metoprolol 25 mg bid, albuterol inhaler 2 puffs 4 times a day as needed as rescue, and suboxone 8 mg/2 mg one film bid. Owing to her housing safety concerns, she decided to stay at her son's apartment that did not have air conditioning and was problematic due to the warm summer weather and high humidity. Additional outpatient referrals included home health, occupational therapy, and physical therapy.

She followed up with her primary care provider the day after discharge. It was noted that she had gained 35 lbs prior to hospitalization. Upon review of Phyllis' medical records from her hospitalization, a diagnosis of heart failure with preserved ejection fraction (HFpEF) was made. Lasix 20 mg daily was initiated and orders for lab work in 1 week were provided to the patient to evaluate her potassium and kidney function. The nurse practitioner also had an end-of-life discussion with Phyllis and her son. Phyllis decided to be a full code.

Several barriers were encountered when Phyllis was discharged home making the transition difficult. As the discharge diagnosis of HFpEF was not included in the medical record, home health was not prepared with the necessary equipment and education needed for a successful discharge. Phyllis' community has limited access to pharmacy services and providers on the weekend. Fortunately, Phyllis was discharged during the week and was evaluated by her provider within 24 hours of discharge. Medication reconciliation proved to be difficult. Phyllis received an inaccurate suboxone prescription during discharge. The provider who usually treated her opioid addiction was out of town. The transitional care NP had to collaborate with another physician that would agree to assume Phyllis' care in her providers absence and prescribe the correct dose of suboxone. A discussion among the transitional care NP, cardiology, and nephrology also ensued to determine whether the use of an angiotensin receptor–neprilysin inhibitor would be utilized for Phyllis' HFpEF. Complicating matters further, the transitional care NP had to obtain prior authorization for the use of the medication by the insurance company. Starter samples were available in the cardiology office; however, the office was located 120 miles away.

A community care team was created to assist with Phyllis' care. In a rural community, enlisting the services of a community care team can be an option to assist with the complexities of care. Volunteers, first responders, or other community services that are available and familiar with the culture of a rural community could be helpful. Local volunteers worked to clean Phyllis' apartment. A local grocery store delivered food and other household items. Laundry facilities were not available; however, a local thrift shop had a stackable washer/dryer unit that was affordable. The transitional care team and home health were able to secure an air conditioner, bedside commode, and other durable medical equipment. Working with the owner of the apartment, law enforcement, and/or social workers could help with resolving the housing challenges until other options were identified.

Cardiac and pulmonary rehab were offered but Phyllis refused. A physical therapist and a respiratory therapist with prior experience in cardiac rehab were assigned to the team and made home visits twice a week. Home health nurses drew blood work as needed and the Department of Health and Human Services workers provided referrals for transportation for local follow-up visits. The outpatient dialysis clinic's staff evaluated Phyllis three times a week for improving kidney function and kept in close contact with her nephrology providers. Adjustments to her treatment were made as needed. A registered dietician and a social worker worked with her weekly. The transitional NP became the chair of her community care team and was responsible for the coordination of her care. Initially, the team met every other week and then monthly dependent on Phyllis' needs.

Practice Pearls

The complexities of this case are commonly seen when providing care to an older adult with complex comorbid conditions. Ideally, direct communication between the discharging provider, the home health agency, the outpatient dialysis clinic, therapists, specialist providers, and the primary care NP should have occurred to ensure coordination of care. A transitional care NP at the hospital could coordinate and collaborate with the inpatient health care team and the outpatient community team. A transitional care team could facilitate communication of needs and provide a controlled and informed discharge and successful transition to home. Communication and teamwork assisted this patient after discharge to be in a healthier state than when she was admitted which did lead to more positive outcomes in this case. It is imperative that nurses and NPs are educated to address the key concepts included in this case and are astute to a patient's needs when providing care. When needs are identified and addressed before discharge, the transition is a much smoother and safer process.

SUMMARY

Older adults are at a higher risk for developing kidney disease due to aging, multiple complex comorbid conditions, polypharmacy, and changes in volume status. Individuals with kidney disease experience an extensive number of transition of care across health care settings related to the kidney disease process and the number of health care providers involved in their care. Kidney disease is multifactorial, and the prevention of progression of disease and poor outcomes are key to improving the health of individuals with kidney disease. Nurses and NPs can improve the outcomes for individuals with complex comorbid conditions and kidney disease especially during the transitions of care. Older adults with complex comorbid conditions, functional and cognitive limitations are at a higher risk for fragmentation of care[25,26] placing them at a higher risk for complications related to kidney disease. Transitional care should be integrated into the delivery of care daily by all nurses and NPs. Nurse and NPs should develop competency and proficiency in transitional care. Ultimately, nurses who are involved in the coordination of care during transitions of care can reduce rehospitalization, health care costs, and enhance the lives of older adults.

CLINICS CARE POINTS

- Naylor's Transitional Care Model is an evidence-based, nurse-led, team-based model utilized to improve the quality of care of individuals during the transitions of care.
- Determining an individual's healthcare goals is a vital component when determining the plan of care.
- Communication between all members of the healthcare team can ensure consistent delivery of the plan of care.

DISCLOSURE

The authors have nothing to disclose.

REFERENCES

1. on Aging Administration. 2020 profile of older Americans. 2021. Available at: https://acl.gov/sites/default/files/Aging%20and%20Disability%20in%20America/2020ProfileOlderAmericans.Final_.pdf. Accessed June 1, 2022.
2. American Association of Colleges of Nursing. Fact sheet: nursing shortage. 2020. Available at: https://www.aacnnursing.org/Portals/42/News/Factsheets/Nursing-Shortage-Factsheet.pdf. Accessed June 1, 2022.
3. of Medicine Institute. The future of nursing: leading change, Advancing Health. 2008. Available at: https://pubmed.ncbi.nlm.nih.gov/24983041/. Accessed June 1, 2022.
4. National Academies of Scienced, Engineering, and Medicine. The future of nursing 2020-2030: charting a path to achieve health equity. Washington, D.C.: The National Academies Press; 2021. https://doi.org/10.17226/25982.
5. Boersma P, Black L. Prevalence of multiple chronic conditions among US adults, 2018. Prev Chronic Dis 2020;17:200130.
6. Kidney Foundation National. Aging and kidney disease. 2022. Available at: https://www.kidney.org/news/monthly/wkd_aging. Accessed June 1, 2022.
7. United States Renal Data System. 2021 annal Data report. 2021. Available at: https://adr.usrds.org/2021. Accessed June 1, 2022.
8. United States Renal Data System. Transition of care in chronic kidney disease. 2019. Available at: https://www.usrds.org/media/2366/usrds-tcckd-2019-report.pdf. Accessed June 1, 2022.

9. Weinhandl ED, Gilbertson DT, Wetmore JB, et al. COVID-19- associated decline in the size of the end-stage kidney disease population in the United States. Kidney Int Rep 2021;6:2698–701.

10. Silver SA, Adhikari NK, Bell CM, et al. Nephrologist follow-up vs. Usual care after an AKI hospitalization (FUSION): a randomized control trial. Clin J Am Soc Neph 2021;16:1005–14.

11. Harding JL, Yanfeng L, Burrows NR, et al. US trends in hospitalizations for dialysis-requiring acute kidney injury in people with vs. without diabetes. Am J Kid Dis 2019;75(6):897–907.

12. Hirschman KB, Shaid E, McCauley K, et al. Continuity of care: the transitional care model. OJIN 2015;20(No. 3). Manuscript 1.

13. Kalantar-Zadeh K, Kovesdy CP, Streja E, et al. Transitions of care from pre-dialysis prelude to renal replacement therapy: the blueprints of emerging research in advanced chronic kidney disease. Nephrol Dial Transpl 2017;32: ii91–8.

14. Evans M, Lopau K. The transitions clinic in chronic kidney disease care. Nephrol Dial Transpl 2020;35:ii4–10.

15. Kidney International. Kidney disease improving global outcomes clinical Practice Guidelines for acute kidney injury. 2012. Available at: https://kdigo.org/guidelines/acute-kidney-injury/. Accessed June 1, 2022.

16. Welch JL, Bartlett Ellis RJ, Ambuehl R, et al. Patterns of healthcare encounters experienced by patients with chronic kidney disease. J Ren Care 2017;43(4): 209–18.

17. Vijayan A, Abdel EM, Liu K, et al. Recovery after critical illness and acute kidney injury. Clin J Am Soc Neph 2021;16:1601–9.

18. Mehta R, Bihorac A, Selby NM, et al, and for the Acute Dialysis Quality Initiative Consensus Group. Establishing a continuum of acute kidney injury- tracing AKI using Data source linkage and long-term follow-up: workgroup statements from the 15th ADQI Consensus conference. Can J Kidney Health Dis 2016;3:1–13.

19. United States Renal Data System. Acute kidney injury. 2020. Available at: https://adr.usrds.org/2020/chronic-kidney-disease/5-acute-kidney-injury.

20. Duronville JV, Diamantidis CJ. Medical safety in the care of the person with end stage kidney disease. Semin Dial 2018;31:140–8.

21. Behnke L, Rivera S, Chaperon C, et al. Transitions of care. Washington, DC: National Organization of Nurse Practitioner Faculty; 2022.

22. Mora K, Dorrejo XM, Carreon KM, et al. Nurse practitioner led transitional care interventions: an integrative review. J Am Acad Nurse Pract 2017;29:773–90.

23. McBryde M, Vandiver JW, Onysko M. Transitions of care in medical education: a compilation of effective teaching methods. Fam Med 2016;48(4):265–72.

24. Blomberg BA, Mulligan RC, Staub SJ, et al. Handing off the older patient: improved documentation of geriatric assessment in transitions of care. J Am Geriatr Soc 2017;66(2):401–6.

25. Ljungholm L, Klinga C, Edin-Liljegren A, et al. What matters in care continuity on the chronic care trajectory for patients and family carers?- A conceptual model. J Clin Nurs 2022;31:1327–38.

26. Mohammad N, DiTommaso M, Jacobsen S. Nurse practitioner led care transitions program: medication management from skilled nursing facility to home. J Nurs Pract 2020;16:560–3.

UNITED STATES POSTAL SERVICE® Statement of Ownership, Management, and Circulation
(All Periodicals Publications Except Requester Publications)

1. Publication Title	2. Publication Number	3. Filing Date
CRITICAL CARE NURSING CLINICS OF NORTH AMERICA	006 – 273	9/18/22

4. Issue Frequency	5. Number of Issues Published Annually	6. Annual Subscription Price
MAR, JUN SEP, DEC	4	$160.00

7. Complete Mailing Address of Known Office of Publication (Not printer) (Street, city, county, state, and ZIP+4®)

ELSEVIER INC.
230 Park Avenue, Suite 800
New York, NY 10169

Contact Person
Malathi Samayan

Telephone (Include area code)
91-44-4299-4507

8. Complete Mailing Address of Headquarters or General Business Office of Publisher (Not printer)

ELSEVIER INC.
230 Park Avenue, Suite 800
New York, NY 10169

9. Full Names and Complete Mailing Addresses of Publisher, Editor, and Managing Editor (Do not leave blank)

Publisher (Name and complete mailing address)

DOLORES MELONI, ELSEVIER INC.
1600 JOHN F KENNEDY BLVD. SUITE 1800
PHILADELPHIA, PA 19103-2899

Editor (Name and complete mailing address)

KERRY HOLLAND, ELSEVIER INC.
1600 JOHN F KENNEDY BLVD. SUITE 1800
PHILADELPHIA, PA 19103-2899

Managing Editor (Name and complete mailing address)

PATRICK MANLEY, ELSEVIER INC.
1600 JOHN F KENNEDY BLVD. SUITE 1800
PHILADELPHIA, PA 19103-2899

10. Owner (Do not leave blank. If the publication is owned by a corporation, give the name and address of the corporation immediately followed by the names and addresses of all stockholders owning or holding 1 percent or more of the total amount of stock. If not owned by a corporation, give the names and addresses of the individual owners. If owned by a partnership or other unincorporated firm, give its name and address as well as those of each individual owner. If the publication is published by a nonprofit organization, give its name and address.)

Full Name	Complete Mailing Address
WHOLLY OWNED SUBSIDIARY OF REED/ELSEVIER, US HOLDINGS	1600 JOHN F KENNEDY BLVD. SUITE 1800 PHILADELPHIA, PA 19103-2899

11. Known Bondholders, Mortgagees, and Other Security Holders Owning or Holding 1 Percent or More of Total Amount of Bonds, Mortgages, or Other Securities. If none, check box ► ☐ None

Full Name	Complete Mailing Address
N/A	

12. Tax Status (For completion by nonprofit organizations authorized to mail at nonprofit rates) (Check one)
The purpose, function, and nonprofit status of this organization and the exempt status for federal income tax purposes:
☒ Has Not Changed During Preceding 12 Months
☐ Has Changed During Preceding 12 Months (Publisher must submit explanation of change with this statement)

PS Form 3526, July 2014 (Page 1 of 4 (see instructions page 4)) PSN: 7530-01-000-9931   PRIVACY NOTICE: See our privacy policy on www.usps.com.

---

13. Publication Title	14. Issue Date for Circulation Data Below
CRITICAL CARE NURSING CLINICS OF NORTH AMERICA	JUNE 2022

15. Extent and Nature of Circulation			Average No. Copies Each Issue During Preceding 12 Months	No. Copies of Single Issue Published Nearest to Filing Date
a. Total Number of Copies (Net press run)			137	112
b. Paid Circulation (By Mail and Outside the Mail)	(1)	Mailed Outside-County Paid Subscriptions Stated on PS Form 3541 (Include paid distribution above nominal rate, advertiser's proof copies, and exchange copies)	78	57
	(2)	Mailed In-County Paid Subscriptions Stated on PS Form 3541 (Include paid distribution above nominal rate, advertiser's proof copies, and exchange copies)	0	0
	(3)	Paid Distribution Outside the Mails Including Sales Through Dealers and Carriers, Street Vendors, Counter Sales, and Other Paid Distribution Outside USPS®	26	25
	(4)	Paid Distribution by Other Classes of Mail Through the USPS (e.g., First-Class Mail®)	0	0
c. Total Paid Distribution (Sum of 15b (1), (2), (3), and (4))		►	104	82
d. Free or Nominal Rate Distribution (By Mail and Outside the Mail)	(1)	Free or Nominal Rate Outside-County Copies included on PS Form 3541	18	16
	(2)	Free or Nominal Rate In-County Copies Included on PS Form 3541	0	0
	(3)	Free or Nominal Rate Copies Mailed at Other Classes Through the USPS (e.g. First-Class Mail)	0	0
	(4)	Free or Nominal Rate Distribution Outside the Mail (Carriers or other means)	0	0
e. Total Free or Nominal Rate Distribution (Sum of 15d (1), (2), (3) and (4))		►	18	16
f. Total Distribution (Sum of 15c and 15e)		►	122	98
g. Copies not Distributed (See Instructions to Publishers #4 (page #3))		►	15	14
h. Total (Sum of 15f and g)		►	137	112
i. Percent Paid (15c divided by 15f times 100)		►	85.24%	83.67%

* If you are claiming electronic copies, go to line 16 on page 3. If you are not claiming electronic copies, skip to line 17 on page 3.

PS Form 3526, July 2014 (Page 2 of 4)

16. Electronic Copy Circulation	Average No. Copies Each Issue During Preceding 12 Months	No. Copies of Single Issue Published Nearest to Filing Date
a. Paid Electronic Copies	►	
b. Total Paid Print Copies (Line 15c) + Paid Electronic Copies (Line 16a)	►	
c. Total Print Distribution (Line 15f) + Paid Electronic Copies (Line 16a)	►	
d. Percent Paid (Both Print & Electronic Copies) (16b divided by 16c × 100)	►	

☒ I certify that 50% of all my distributed copies (electronic and print) are paid above a nominal price.

17. Publication of Statement of Ownership

☒ If the publication is a general publication, publication of this statement is required. Will be printed   ☐ Publication not required.
in the DECEMBER 2022 issue of this publication.

18. Signature and Title of Editor, Publisher, Business Manager, or Owner

Malathi Samayan

Malathi Samayan - Distribution Controller

Date   9/18/22

I certify that all information furnished on this form is true and complete. I understand that anyone who furnishes false or misleading information on this form or who omits material or information requested on the form may be subject to criminal sanctions (including fines and imprisonment) and/or civil sanctions (including civil penalties).

PS Form 3526, July 2014 (Page 3 of 4)   PRIVACY NOTICE: See our privacy policy on www.usps.com.

Moving?

Make sure your subscription moves with you!

To notify us of your new address, find your **Clinics Account Number** (located on your mailing label above your name), and contact customer service at:

Email: journalscustomerservice-usa@elsevier.com

800-654-2452 (subscribers in the U.S. & Canada)
314-447-8871 (subscribers outside of the U.S. & Canada)

Fax number: 314-447-8029

**Elsevier Health Sciences Division
Subscription Customer Service
3251 Riverport Lane
Maryland Heights, MO 63043**

*To ensure uninterrupted delivery of your subscription, please notify us at least 4 weeks in advance of move.

Printed and bound by CPI Group (UK) Ltd, Croydon, CR0 4YY

03/10/2024

01040466-0013